REFRACTIVE SURGERY: A TEXT OF RADIAL KERATOTOMY

Edited By
Donald R. Sanders MD, PhD
Robert F. Hofmann MD

Printed in the United States of America

Library of Congress Catalog Card Number: 84-51816

ISBN: 0-943432-34-0

Published by: SLACK Incorporated
               6900 Grove Rd.
               Thorofare, NJ 08086

Last digit is print number: 10   9   8   7   6   5   4   3   2   1

CONTRIBUTING AUTHORS

Jerome W. Bettman, M.D.
Emeritus Clinical Professor
Pacific Medical Center;
Stanford University; and
University of California at San Francisco

Warren D. Cross, M.D.
Chief of Ophthalmology
12 Oaks Hospital
Houston

Michael R. Deitz, M.D.
Clinical Assistant Professor
University of Missouri
Kansas City

Robert E. Fenzl, M.D., F.A.C.S.
Assistant Clinical Professor
University of California, Irvine, CA
Director of the Orange County Eye Bank

William Justus Head III, M.D.
12 Oaks Hospital
Houston
Institute of Eye Surgery
Houston

Robert F. Hofmann, M.D.
Mercy Hospital, Denver
Porter Memorial Hospital
Denver

G. William Lavery, M.D.
Clinical Instructor
University of Texas at Houston
Northeast Medical Center Hospital
Humble

Andrew O. Lewicky, M.D., F.A.C.S.
Assistant Professor of Ophthalmology
Rush Medical College
Associate Ophthalmologist
Rush Presbyterian St. Luke's Medical Center
Attending Ophthalmologist
Michael Reese Medical Center and Grant Hospital of Chicago

Richard L. Lindstrom, M.D.
Assistant Professor of Ophthalmology
Department of Ophthalmology
University of Minnesota
Minneapolis

William Myers, M.D.
Director of the Michigan Eye Institute
Southfield
Assistant Clinical Professor
Michigan State University
Lansing

James J. Salz, M.D.
Associate Clinical Professor
Ophthalmology
University of Southern California

Donald R. Sanders, M.D., Ph.D.
Associate Professor of Ophthalmology
University of Illinois Eye and Ear Infirmary
Chief of Ophthalmology
West Side Veterans Hospital
Chicago

Spencer P. Thornton, M.D., F.A.C.S.
Chief, Department of Ophthalmology
Baptist Hospital
Nashville
Director, Cataract and Corneal Surgery Service
Director, Surgical Research
Eye Foundation of Tennessee

Richard A. Villasenor, M.D.
Associate Clinical Professor of Ophthalmology
Dohenny Eye Foundation
University of Southern California
Director
Holy Cross Hospital Refractive Surgery

CONTENTS

ACKNOWLEDGMENTS

No work of this dimension can be completed without the assistance and contributions of many individuals "behind the scenes." The editors and contributors wish to acknowledge the quiet contributions of their staff personnel who provide a smooth office environment at all times, and particularly as publishing deadlines approach for the authors.

We also wish to acknowledge the creative contributions of Jayn C. Montgomery, Littleton, Colorado and Nancy Snyder, Chicago, Illinois for special medical illustrations and Donald Radcliffe, Chicago, for editorial assistance with the manuscripts.

The support of our respective medical centers and ophthalmology institutions is also critical and greatly appreciated. I (DRS) particularly wish to thank my department chairman, Dr. Morton Goldberg, for his continuing support of my research. On a personal note, the editors wish to thank our wives, Wanda Sanders and Geraldine Hofmann, for their forbearance and patience during this project.

Donald R. Sanders, M.D., Ph.D.
Robert Hofmann, M.D.

PREFACE

The quest for a method to correct refractive errors through a precise and safe surgical procedure has been under way for nearly half a century. The attempts to modify the curvature of the anterior surface of the cornea have focused on two methods: 1) incisional relaxation, and 2) lathing. In this book, we will consider the techniques currently being used in incisional refractive keratoplasty.

The history of incisional techniques to correct refractive errors has been riddled with controversy on the one hand and marked by brilliant scientific inquiry on the other hand. The controversy centers less on the science of corneal surface modification and more on the philosophical question of whether one should attempt to change a so-called "healthy cornea."

It is true that the cornea of a patient with myopia or astigmatism is not technically pathologic. Nonetheless, the refractive state of that patient's eye causes "dis"ease to the patient, despite the use of prosthetic devices to correct for the refractive error. In this light, one's philosophy of the nature of a healthy cornea may be modified somewhat when one actually performs incisional refractive surgery such as radial keratotomy (RK). At the same time, however, the goal of all ophthalmic surgery—better vision for the patient—remains the same.

As these techniques in refractive surgery evolve, their eventual goal is to improve the well-being of patients by eliminating or minimizing visual "dis"ease as well as ocular disease. Although the full impact of the successful evolution of incisional refractive surgery has yet to be realized, many persons who have been hindered by a genetic defect from their fullest visual potential now can look forward to the day when the limitations will no longer be present.

This textbook is intended to be a treatise on current clinical techniques in radial keratotomy and its analogues for the correction of myopia and astigmatism. It is as complete and authoritative as a work can be in a field that is still evolving, and evolution is very much a characteristic of the present field of refractive surgery.

Radial keratotomy has really existed as a widely used procedure for only a dozen years, and in the next decades, it will be facing further development and refinement. Not all the answers are yet known about radial keratotomy and its analogues. In truth, not all the questions have yet been asked.

This text is a compendium of knowledge from experienced academic as well as private practice surgeons who are expert in the field of refractive keratoplasty. It is an. honor as well as a privilege to present the work, philosophy, and insights of the contributors to this book. We hope that this text will bring to the field of refractive keratoplasty a closer examination, greater understanding, and deserved acceptance by the ophthalmic community.

Donald R. Sanders, M.D., Ph.D.
Robert F. Hofmann, M.D.

Chapter 1

The History of Radial Keratotomy

Richard A. Villaseñor, MD

THE HISTORY OF RADIAL KERATOTOMY

Radial keratotomy is the most controversial ophthalmic surgery performed today, and yet it is potentially a very beneficial procedure for a select group of patients. This dichotomy is of long standing. For nearly two hundred years, ophthalmic surgeons have been attempting to correct refractive errors by surgical means. The roster of major contributors to the various forms of refractive surgery, including radial keratotomy, is noteworthy.[1]

Since this book deals exclusively with radial keratotomy, the history described here begins appropriately with Sato's works. His early investigations began in 1939 and were published in 1953.[2] The initial work was intended for the correction of keratoconus rather than for myopia.[3] By inducing surgical hydrops through endothelial incisions directly under an eccentric cone, significant flattening of the keratoconus occurred after several weeks of patching (Figure 1-1). Kanai, who is following Sato's patients at the University of Juntendo in Tokyo, is still moderately enthusi-

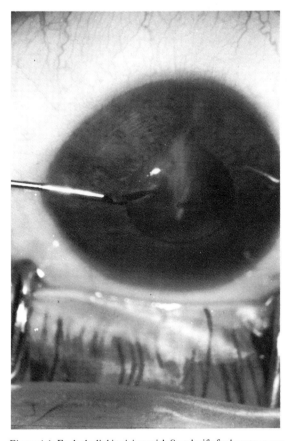

Figure 1-1: Endothelial incision with Sato knife for keratoconus correction.

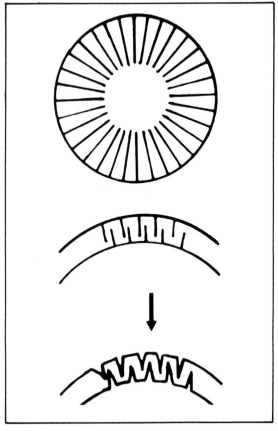

Figure 1-2: Multiple corneal incisions were made both on the anterior and posterior surfaces of the cornea.

astic about this procedure, but negative about posterior radial keratotomy for congenital myopia.

Sato's work with keratoconus ultimately led him to the correction of astigmatism and then to the correction of congenital myopia. He began by making as many as 32 incisions on the anterior surface of the cornea, and eventually entered the anterior chamber to make 32 or more additional incisions on the endothelial surface in order to achieve a greater correction, (Figure 1-2). In spite of these multiple incisions and a constant 6.0 mm optic zone, he still only obtained an average of 3 diopters of correction.

While the technique appeared successful for many years, a high percentage of these corneas eventually decompensated. As many as 80% of the cases followed at Juntendo University have ultimately undergone corneal decompensation (Figure 1-3). This is particularly significant since it occurred in a population in which endothelial corneal dystrophy is virtually unknown. Nearly all of the cases decompensated at about 40 years of age, irrespective of the patient's age at the time of operation (Table 1-1).

Penetrating keratoplasty on this group of patients was not initially successful (Figure 1-4). In 1976, seven grafts were attempted with a zero success rate (Table 1-2). In a second series, the success rate improved, with five out of 12 cases being considered successful (Table 1-2).

It is believed that the poor success rate was not due to something inherent in the rejected cornea, but rather to the poor quality of donor tissue available in Japan. Religious beliefs in Japan proscribe tissue donation for transplantation. The corneas were actually obtained from Sri Lanka, a small island located south of India where poor transportation and less than optimal tissue handling probably contributed to the graft failures. On the other hand, Steiner[4] recently performed a penetrating keratoplasty on a complicated case of radial keratotomy in the United States with an excellent result.

Credit for the current interest and success of radial keratotomy must go to S.N. Fyodorov[5] of Russia. He reported his initial series in 1979, arousing tremendous interest in the United States. In a group of patients with 1 to 3

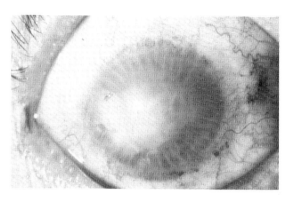

Figure 1-3: Corneal decompensation 20 years following radial keratotomy by Sato.

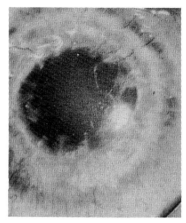

Figure 1-4: Penetrating keratoplasty failure following radial keratotomy.

Table 1-1.
Time Course of Appearance of Bullous Keratopathy Related to Patient Age at Time of Sato Procedure

	Age at Time of Sato Procedure (A)	Patient Age at Appearance of Bullous Keratopathy (B)	Interval Between Sato Procedure and Appearance of Bullous Keratopathy (B-A)
Myopia	14-19 years old	40.0 years old	24.0 years
	20-24 years old	42.0 years old	20.0 years
	25-30 years old	41.0 years old	14.0 years
Myopic Astigmatism	19-34 years old	43.7 years old	19.3 years

Table 1-1: The Age of Surgery; The Age at Which Bullous Keratopathy Occurred; Years Prior to Keratopathy.

Table 1-2.
Results of Penetrating Keratoplasty After the Sato Procedure

Number of Penetrating Keratoplasties		Number of Clear Grafts
-1976	7	0
1977-1980	12	5

Table 1-2: 0% Success Rate in 1976 Improving to Nearly 50% in the Next Series.

diopters of myopia preoperatively, he reported that 100% of the patients obtained visual acuities of 20/50 or better without correction, and 85% were 20/25 or better.

The next report was from Bores[6] of the United States who presented his initial results in 1980 and began offering the first instructional courses in radial keratotomy. He volunteered to help design the protocol for the Prospective Evaluation of Radial Keratotomy (PERK) study which is funded by the National Institutes of Health and coordinated by George Waring, M.D.[7]

Eight university centers across the United States participated in this study, each performing 50 cases. The study was designed so that all surgeons performed the surgery as similarly as possible. Instructional courses and proctors during surgery helped to achieve uniformity of surgery. Independent monitors recorded the postoperative results and forwarded them to the collecting center for computer analysis.

The data from the PERK study are still pending, but the initial reports were scheduled to be made available at the 1984 American Academy of Ophthalmology meeting in Atlanta. While it will be several years before all of the data are released, it is my impression that the study will suggest that, when it is performed properly, radial keratotomy is a safe and effective procedure for correction of myopia.

The technique of radial keratotomy has evolved considerably since its first introduction by Fyodorov. Optical pachymetry for measuring the corneal thickness has been replaced, for the most part, by ultrasonic pachymetry. The metal blade fragments have been replaced with diamond knives with micrometer handles. These two advances have markedly decreased the complication rate and increased predictability. The initial 16 incisions, recommended by Fyodorov, have now been reduced to eight incisions. Schachar,[8] in his theoretical model of the eye, predicted that eight incisions would be 90% as effective as 16, as did Knauss and Smith[9,10] of the Estelle Doheny Eye Foundation, on a similar corneal model designed by the Massachusetts Institute of Technology. Salz[11] confirmed this observation later in bank eyes. Myers[12] subsequently presented the first human data on eight radial incisions, confirming all the theoretical data, and significantly contributing to the modification to eight incisions. The results of radial keratotomy from the University of California at Los Angeles' second series again confirmed these findings.[13]

While eight incisions are most commonly performed today, there is a tendency toward even fewer incisions. Salz and Villaseñor[14] presented their results on the further modification to four incisions for the correction of low to moderate degrees of myopia, and they advocate this technique.

There is no standard method of performing radial keratotomy at the present time. Techniques are nearly as variable as the number of surgeons performing the procedure. This is unfortunate because it will necessitate a longer period of time in which to predict the variables. While radial keratotomy is generally considered safe, certain techniques performed today undeniably cannot be considered safe. Multiple reoperations are to be viewed with extreme caution. Endothelial cell loss has been documented at 3% to 10% with each surgery.[13,15] There are several publications on the results of radial keratotomy which include the work of the ARK (Analysis of Radial Keratotomy) Study Group,[16] Bores,[17] Rowsey,[18] Fyodorov,[19] Cowden,[20] Deitz,[21] Hoffer,[13] and others. All of the authors confirm that the surgery is effective in reducing myopia in the 1 to 6 diopter range, but their technique, for the most part, is generally varied.

Today in the United States, radial keratotomy is being performed in virtually every major city, and approximately 90,000 cases have been done in all. The number of surgeries performed is increasing and will continue to do so unless major complications appear. Numerous investigators are working on methods that promise, barring major problems, to improve markedly the accuracy of the procedure. There are several variables now that appear to have definite effects on the surgical outcome; these will be mentioned later in this book.

Computer software has been developed in which the surgeon enters the major variables and the recommended surgery is printed out. At least one of these programs recommends redeepening and the use of 16 incisions, a technique that is questioned by many. Currently, most refractive surgeons who are doing a large number of cases rely solely on their personal experience and use variables that are particular to themselves. There is research into the use of newer blade materials that are less fragile; sharper metal blades; the use of lasers for making incisions, not only for radial keratotomy but also for keratomileusis; and collagen shrinkage. The newest and one of the most exciting advances is the Ruiz procedure for the correction of large amounts of astigmatism.[22] It can be applied to either congenital, post-cataract, post-penetrating keratoplasty, or post-refractive keratoplasty astigmatism, with the ability to obtain corrections of up to 8 diopters of cylinder.

Refractive surgery as an entity, including all of its various forms, is in an early stage of development, similar to the status of intraocular lenses in 1972. The ophthalmic surgeon should retain a cautious but inquisitive eye on this new surgical field. Sato's early work should *not* be looked upon as a failure, but rather as a steppingstone to the observations of Fyodorov and, ultimately, to the advances that have been made by other investigators. To the degree that the last decade has been known in ophthalmology as the "Decade of the Intraocular Lens," I believe that this one will be known as the "Decade of Refractive Surgery." In the near future, surgical correction of refractive errors will be an acceptable alternative to the use of conventional optical devices.

References

1. Villaseñor RA: Introduction To and Historical Overview of Surgical Procedures for the Correction of Refractive Errors. *In* PS Binder (ed) International Ophthalmic Clinics, Little, Brown and Co, 23:3, Fall 1983. pp 1-9.
2. Sato T, Akiyama K, Shibata H: A New Surgical Approach to Myopia. *Am J Ophthal* 36:823-829, 1953.
3. Sato T: Treatment of Conical Cornea (incision of Descemet's membrane). *Nippon Ganka Gakkai Sasshi*, 43:541, 1939.
4. Steiner GA, Shaw EL, Binder PS, et al.: The Histopathology of a Case of Radial Keratotomy. *Arch Ophthalmol* 100:1473, 1982.
5. Fyodorov SN, Durnev VV: Operation of Dosaged Dissection of Corneal Circular Ligament in Cases of Myopia of Mild Degree. *Ann Ophthalmol* 11:1185-1890, 1979.
6. Bores LD, Myers WD, Deitz MD (independent reports): National Radial Keratotomy Study Group Course. Santa Monica Hospital, Los Angeles, May 1980.
7. Waring GO III: Radial Keratotomy in Perspective. *Ophthal Forum* 1:12-14, 1982.
8. Schachar RA, Black TD, Huang T: A Mathematical Model for Radial Keratotomy. *In* Understanding Radial Keratotomy, LAL Publ: Denison TX, pp 12-18, 1981.
9. Knauss W, Rapacz P, Sene K: Curvature Changes Induced by Radial Keratotomy in Solithane Model of Eye. *Invest Ophthalmol Vis Sci* (ARVO abstracts) 20(Suppl):69, 1982.
10. Smith RE, Luttrull JK, Jester JV: The Effect of Radial Keratotomy on Ocular Integrity in an Animal Model. *Arch Ophthalmol* 100:319, 1982.
11. Salz JJ, Lee J, Jester J, Steel DL, Villaseñor RA, Nesburn A, Smith RE: Radial Keratotomy in Fresh Human Cadaver Eyes. *Ophthalmol (Rochester)* 88:742, 1981.
12. Myers WD: The Evolution of Radial Keratotomy. *In* RA Schachar, NS Levy, L Schachar (eds) Radial Keratotomy, LAL Pub: Denison, TX, pp 67-89, 1980.
13. Hoffer R, Levenson JE: UCLA Clinical Trial of Radial Keratotomy. *Ophthalmol (Rochester)* 88:729, 1981.
14. Salz JJ, Villaseñor RA: Clinical Results of Four Incision Radial Keratotomy. Keratorefractive Society Meeting, Chicago, IL, November, 1983.
15. Smith RE, Jester JV, Arthur JB, Salz JJ, Steel DL: Endothelial Studies Following Radial Keratotomy in Primate Eyes. *Invest Ophthalmol* (Suppl) 22(3):240, 1982.
16. Sanders, D (ed): *Radial Keratotomy: ARK Study Group*, Thorofare, NJ: Slack Publications, 1984.
17. Bores LD, Myers WD, Cowden J: Radial Keratotomy: An analysis of the American experience. *Ann Ophthalmol* 13:941-948, 1981.
18. Rowsey JJ and Balyeat HD: Preliminary Results and Complications of Radial Keratotomy. *Am J Ophthalmol* 93:437, 1982.
19. Fyodorov S: Surgical Correction of Myopia and Astigmatism. *In* RA Schachar, NS Levy, and L Schachar (eds), Keratorefraction, Denison, TX: LAL Publ., 1980, pp 141-170.

20. Cowden JW: Radial Keratotomy: a Retrospective Study of Cases Observed at the Kresge Eye Institute for Six Months. *Arch Ophthalmol* 100:578-580, 1982.
21. Deitz M, Sanders DR, Marks R: Radial Keratotomy: An Overview of the Kansas City Study. *Ophthalmology* 91(5):467-477, 1984.
22. Nordan LT: *Current Status of Refractive Surgery.* San Diego, CA: CL Printing, 1983, pp 13-30.

Chapter 2

Refractive Keratoplasty: Medicolegal Aspects

Jerome W. Bettman, MD

REFRACTIVE KERATOPLASTY: MEDICOLEGAL ASPECTS

In the present milieu of frequent litigation it is important for surgeons to consider the risk of medicolegal involvement when performing newer procedures such as refractive keratoplasty. Elective procedures carry a greater medicolegal hazard than those that are required or are without better alternatives. This hazard varies with the benefits and risks of the procedure compared with alternative ones. Consider, for example, the case of a surgeon who does an epikeratoplasty in an aphakic patient who is unable to wear spectacles or contact lenses and in whom the alternative would be a secondary lens implant. This surgeon could present a very strong case that epikeratoplasty is less hazardous than the alternative.

On the other hand, a radial keratotomy performed on a patient who simply does not wish to wear spectacles presents a much greater hazard. The expected benefit is to dispense with spectacles of moderate strength, but even this benefit cannot be assured. Some complications are not too serious and are well known; these include glare if the incisions are within the pupillary area; uncertainty of the resulting refraction; and variable refraction for a period of time. These complications may be tolerable, but more serious complications may be a threat to vision or to the eye itself. These catastrophies include the possibility of endophthalmitis following perforation as well as long-term hazards such as blunt trauma to the weakened peripheral cornea; possible corneal decompensation; and others. The latter present a serious threat of lawsuits.

Patients who are intolerant of relatively minor inconvenience, such as wearing spectacles, are the type of persons who are more likely to sue than are more phlegmatic types. The expectations of intolerant types of patients are high, and there is room for disappointment. The disappointed patient may become angry, and anger may result in a suit.

There are occasions when the need for radial keratotomy is greater than the alternatives, as in the case of an airline pilot who can no longer pass the physical examination because of increasing myopia; but even this situation is not without hazard. I have reviewed such a case in which there was a perforation during the procedure, followed by endophthalmitis, loss of the eye, and loss of occupation as well.

With the exception of the last case, this chapter is not based upon actual cases, for two reasons: 1) these procedures have not been done in very large numbers until recently, and there must be a large base of procedures to provide a significant number of claims; and 2) there is a long delay from the time a procedure is done until it comes to adjudication. Other than the theoretical considerations, I know of no way to estimate the incidence of claims in the future.

The need for fully informed consent is geometrically greater in elective procedures. In cases of refractive keratoplasty fully informed consent is of the greatest importance from both legal and ethical standpoints. There are several aspects of informed consent that are important. The use of printed forms is acceptable, in part, and may be required. It is of utmost importance to realize, however, that printed forms, brochures, tapes, or movies are never a substitute for personal exchange between surgeon and patient. If one uses a prepared or packaged method of informed consent as indicated, the surgeon should always follow up by asking patients if they understand what they read and if there are any questions; the surgeon should also obtain some "feedback" to be certain patients do understand. Patients will frequently read a consent form and sign it because—in their words—"the doctor wouldn't have asked me to sign it if it weren't proper that it be done," or "I don't really know what this means, but I'd better sign it and not cause a delay in this busy office."

The timing of informed consent is also very significant. A patient who is about to enter the hospital or who is in the hospital is frequently concerned about the admission procedure and will sign a document without careful thought. A document signed under these circumstances is meaningless and conveys nothing regarding truly informed consent. An attorney representing the patient later can present such situations to a jury with some drama, and the significance of a mere signature on a document can be nullified. I believe that a minimal procedure should also include a note in the surgeon's own hand as follows: "The procedure, the complications, the alternatives, and the anesthetic risks were explained to (patient's name) and (he or she) appeared to understand." This is of significance because a jury reasons that the surgeon took the trouble to write the note and therefore probably did inform the patient, whereas a printed form may have been handed to a patient by any employee and signed without the patient truly understanding it.

In certain cases in which the threat of a lawsuit is great, the surgeon may elect to use a method that the patient cannot dispute: Inform the patient by any means desired, then ask questions to insure that it is all understood. Next, hand the patient his own chart and tell him to write on it what he does understand. If there are any misunderstandings, these should be rewritten by the patient. This documentation cannot be denied! It was written by the patient in his own hand.

The matter of informed consent is important, but there are limits to its importance. Attorneys usually do not like to try cases solely on this complaint. The reason is that trials are conducted years after the operation. By this time the patient and the surgeon have differing or even opposite recollections of what was said, and juries tend to believe the physician. The plaintiff's attorney must also be able to show that the information which was omitted would have caused the patient to have refused to have the procedure performed. The jury will be asked to decide if a prudent person informed of this peril would have declined the procedure. In addition, patients generally do not remember much of what they were told, and only a very few would recall being told of a complication that might result in loss of sight of the eyeball. Physicians interested in the amazing lack of patients' recall should consult the articles by Priluck et al.,[1] Robinson and Misio,[2] and Leeb et al.[3] It is particularly useful to be able to cite these references in instances in which a patient claims that he was not informed of a given risk when the surgeon knows it was discussed.

Is informed consent so very important then in the light of the facts that plaintiffs' attorneys rarely wish to base their claims exclusively on lack of informed consent, and that it can be demonstrated that patients do not recall being told of a majority of the more serious complications? The answer is emphatically "yes." A patient who is fully informed rarely sues. Indeed, there is probably nothing as important in reducing the incidence of lawsuits as taking the patient into your confidence in the decision-making process.

Other factors that are important in reducing incidence of suits, in addition to full and open communication, are a pleasant and properly trained receptionist, good records, and early consultation when indicated.[4] The receptionist should not only be pleasant but be trained to recognize possible emergencies and to keep a record of cancellations and compliance failures on the patient's chart. Good records are essential because they are written at the time of the occurrence and are not subject to the fallacies of memory. A record should never be altered in such a way that the scratched-out material cannot be read, nor should anything ever be added after a claim is filed. Such changes can usually be detected and then the case becomes indefensible.[5] In the event that consultation may be indicated, the surgeon should suggest it before the patient asks for one. The surgeon can then usually pick the consultant, and this is important. The patient's respect generally increases when the surgeon suggests the consultation first.

Adequate insurance coverage is essential to cover this type of surgery. The amount of coverage should certainly be no less than $1,000,000 per event and $3,000,000 per year. There have not been many awards greater than $1,000,000 in ophthalmology. Most huge awards are assessed against more than one defendant: the surgeon, the hospital, and the anesthesiologist, for example.

It might be prudent for the surgeon to carry even more coverage in certain circumstances, such as the following: 1) In some states the statute of limitations runs from the time the patient first becomes aware that his problem might have been caused by substandard care; this might be many years later in the case of a child. 2) The size of awards has increased over the years; consequently the amount of coverage that might be considered adequate at the time of operation might be inadequate if a claim is made a number of years after the alleged substandard event took place. 3) Late complications such as corneal decompensation can occur long after the operation and result in a lawsuit years later, possibly with an even higher award.

Both medicolegal and ethical considerations can almost always be resolved by doing what is in the best interest of the patient without regard for finances, personal aggrandizement, or other possible benefits to the surgeon. Refractive keratoplasty is relatively new, but the legal and ethical approach of always carefully assessing, in all honesty, the benefits and potential risks, both long-term and short-term, is not new. This approach is, however, of increased importance. A surgeon who has honestly weighed the risks and benefits, has always been guided by them, has always communicated freely with his patient, and has welcomed additional opinions need have less concern with the law and ethics than others who do not take these actions. The technical advances in refractive keratoplasty have been astounding and great changes have taken place in the past few years, but human nature has not changed. Honesty, rapport, good records, having consultations when indicated, and always doing what is in the patient's best interests remain and always will remain the fundamentals of good medical practice.

References
1. Priluck I, et al.: What Patients Recall of the Preoperative Discussion after Retinal Detachment Surgery. *Am J Ophthal* 87:620-623, 1979.
2. Robinson G, Merav A: Informed Consent: Recall by patients tested postoperatively. *Am Coll of Surgeons Bulletin* 62:7, 1977.
3. Leeb D, et al.: Observations on the Myth of "Informed Consent." *Plastic and Reconstructive Surgery* 58:280, 1976.
4. Bettman J: *Ophthalmology: The Art, The Law, and a Bit of Science.* Birmingham, AL: Aesculapius Pub Co, pp 10-20.
5. Bettman J, Tennenhouse D: Medicolegal Aspects of Ophthalmology. *Internat Ophthal Clin* 20:4, 1980, Boston, MA: Little Brown & Co, pp 33-42.

Chapter 3

Patient Selection and Counseling

Michael R. Deitz, MD

PATIENT SELECTION AND COUNSELING

The decision to undergo a radial keratotomy procedure is a major and very personal one, perhaps the most important medical decision the patient has ever made. In most medical problems, the physician examines the situation and decides the best course of action, which he or she then recommends to the patient. The patient either complies with the recommendation or seeks another opinion.

Since there is no medical indication for radial keratotomy, however, the physician has no basis on which to make such a determination for the patient. The decision of the risks versus the benefits, the so-called risk-benefit ratio, must lie with the patient. The physician's job is to educate; to counsel; and to make sure the patient is fully aware of the advantages and expected benefits versus the disadvantages, shortcomings, and possible risks of the surgery. The physician must also screen the patient to determine if he is a good candidate for the surgery, both in terms of his refractive needs and his general health, as well as to determine his psychologic suitability for surgery.

This chapter will discuss:
- two general approaches to patient counseling and selection;
- methods of patient counseling and important points to be covered; and
- criteria for patient selection; psychological and physical.

Approaches to Patient Counseling

Unaided 20/20 vision might seem to be the singular, logical goal of any radial keratotomy procedure. However, as important as 20/20 can be, *patient satisfaction* is the real "bottom line" for this or any procedure whose principal justification is improved quality of life. It is quite possible to have 20/20 vision and a dissatisfied patient at the same time. Conversely, many radial keratotomy (RK) patients with less than 20/20 vision can be unbelievably ecstatic about their results. Patient satisfaction demands that their realistic expectations be met or exceeded. To realize this goal, patient counseling must help the patient adopt realistic expectations, the operative parameters must be carefully chosen and the surgery deftly enough performed so the results meet or exceed those expectations.

The physician has at his disposal two general approaches to the problem of patient counseling and selection. These approaches are: 1) to educate groups and then select specific candidates; or 2) to select and then educate specific patients. The author uses a slightly modified version of the 'educate and then select' method. Patients are scheduled for a general public seminar in groups of approximately 15 prospective patients after a brief telephone screening by the office staff. During this screening, patients are eliminated who have obvious contraindications to the surgery such as

Table 3-1
Expected Findings After Radial Keratotomy
With Different Degrees of Myopia*

Preoperative Myopia	Mild 1-3 Diopters	Moderate 3-6 Diopters	Severe 6-10 Diopters
Proportion of First KC Series	15%	60%	25%
% Achieving 20/20	65%	42%	24%
% Achieving 20/40 or better	97%	87%	70%
% ±1 Diopter of Emmetropia	71%	64%	44%
Star Pattern Flare	None, or Occ. Slight	Mild, or Occ. Moderate	Moderate, or Occ. Severe
Fluctuation	Rare	Mild to Moderate	Moderate
16 Cuts and/or Recutting	Very Rare	Infrequent	Common
Perforation	Very Rare	Infrequent	Frequent
Irregular Mires on Keratometry	Essentially None	Rare	Occasional

* Table based on results of first series of 290 cases from Kansas City Study (Ophthalmology 91:467, 1984)

hyperopia, known eye disease, or refractive problems that cannot be corrected with glasses or contact lenses. Patients are advised to bring a copy of their prescription and, if possible, to wear their corrective spectacle lenses.

The seminar consists of a videotape covering the nature of radial keratotomy: its history, performance, and a general review of expected results. It should contain a detailed statement of the risks and complications as specifically outlined in the informed consent. After viewing the videotape, prospective patients are given an opportunity to talk with individuals who have had the surgery, and then the selection process is started. The physician or a member of the staff reviews the patient's degree of myopia (mild, moderate or severe) (Table 3-1). The patient's age, sex, professional or occupational requirements, automatic keratometry reading, and achieved visual acuity, both corrected and uncorrected, are noted. The patient is told whether he appears to be a good candidate or not, and if his correction is within the scope and capacity of radial keratotomy to correct. A fogging technique is shown to the patient in which his eyes are corrected with 50%, 75%, 90%, and 100% of full myopic correction. This demonstrates that radial keratotomy is not precise and does not always produce uncorrected vision as good as the patient's best corrected vision. The patient is then asked if he has any questions. He is assured he may take as long as he wishes to decide about surgery. It is explained that his next step is an appointment for a complete work-up. Using the other approach, some physicians prefer to screen the patients before the videotape and the education process is begun. This method works well if the patient education room is small and facilities for large seminar programs are not available.

General Considerations

Functional Improvement. A common misconception is that radial keratotomy is a cosmetic procedure. RK surgeons who have even a modest experience with the technique know this is not the case. Candidates for RK surgery are acutely aware—or should be informed—that *function* is the most important consideration. While patients may be aware of this fact, many family members and others in the community, who may be a part of the decision-making process, are not so clear about this distinction. Patients sense that while glasses and contact lenses do compensate for their myopic error, they are not a cure. Radial keratotomy, on the other hand, when it is successful, appears to be a true cure. To make this point, analogies have been used which include the way in which surgery eliminates the need for a hearing aid, and the way orthopedic surgery eliminates the need for a walking brace. Obviously, these are parallels to radial keratotomy in that the function of an organ is restored. The device is able to compensate, perhaps quite adequately before surgery, but the surgery restores function and thus achieves a cure. It is true most people do not find glasses or contact lenses as burdensome as leg braces or hearing aids. However, the analogy is accurate and helps to establish the fact that this is truly functional surgery.

Professional or Occupational Requirements. While representing a significant but distinct minority of the patients who have sought radial keratotomy in our office, a professional subgroup of those interested in RK surgery is composed of law enforcement officers, firemen, pilots, and locomotive engineers. These patients most commonly seek RK surgery as a means of enhancing and improving their employment status. It is important that pilots and engineers, particularly, understand that *20/20 is not always the end result of radial keratotomy.* While improvement is desirable and almost certain, perfect vision cannot be guaranteed.

Graduate engineers appear to be the most demanding and the most concerned with some of the shortcomings and drawbacks that others find only to be minor. These professionals should be carefully counseled that ghost images, double vision, glare, and fluctuating vision can be and frequently are, undesirable results of radial keratotomy. While these minor complications improve with time, and the great majority of patients do not find them to be a major problem, it is the engineer who most often appears to be concerned with them. Nevertheless engineers seem to achieve as good an overall result with the surgery, and the same high percentage of them desire to have surgery on the second eye.

Methods of Patient Education. Lectures, booklets, videotapes, and question-and-answer sessions are all being used to educate patients regarding the risks and benefits of radial keratotomy:

Lectures. A lecture can be conducted by the physician or by members of his staff. This is a useful method of reaching groups, especially in hospital and industry settings. The obvious disadvantage is the large time commitment required.

Booklets. Booklets should contain a summary of all the material presented on the videotape. They are a permanent record and are frequently passed on to other prospective patients.

Videotapes. Videotapes can be obtained from several commercial sources, which do a satisfactory job of patient education. However, several physicians actively engaged in radial keratotomy prefer to use a videotape of their own design. While the commercial tapes may establish the background and give a good audiovisual presentation of the scientific facts concerning radial keratotomy, they do not establish or augment the physician-patient relationship. A tape in which the individual surgeon conducts some of the question and answer periods, discusses the office routine the patient will experience, and which is filmed in the physician's own office will give prospective patients an idea of whether they feel comfortable in this setting and working with this particular doctor. The doctor's concern for both the patient's well-being and the quality of their results can be transmitted by such a tape. By the time the physician actually meets the patient, the patient will know if he thinks he will be comfortable placing himself in the care of this doctor. Obviously, the doctor's own results must be described, and any particular areas of concern or danger that he feels should be emphasized can be stressed; these might not receive enough attention in a commercial tape.

The videotape explains why radial keratotomy is desirable, and it should include at least a brief historical background and some documentation of the expected benefits such as: the percentage of patients who have achieved 20/20 and 20/40 vision, and how many might expect to be relieved of the need of wearing glasses. The risks and shortcomings of the procedure can accurately and thoroughly be covered by a detailed description of the informed consent. The most commonly used informed consent is a paraphrasing of the popular intraocular lens informed consent format.

Question and Answer Sessions. A useful idea is to have the patient write down any questions that they may have during the videotape. Once these questions have been answered, the patient is then asked to sign the question and answer sheet showing that he has seen the videotape and has had an opportunity to ask all the questions. These records are permanently stored because patient counseling is an important part of a *bona fide* informed consent.

Informed Consent. After an introduction, the informed consent describes the prosthetic alternatives to radial keratotomy such as glasses, contact lenses, and orthokeratology. It then delineates the risks and problems. Foremost is the danger of an infective organism invading the eye. The patient is informed that if the infection cannot be controlled with antibiotics, the eye could be totally lost. Second is the importance of pointing out that if the scarring is irregular because the cornea does not heal properly, irregular astigmatism could require the use of eyeglasses. It might be of sufficient degree that neither contact lenses or glasses could restore preoperative acuity. It is important to mention that marked undercorrections can occur. While they compose less than 1% of our cases, patients with less than 50% of their preoperative myopia corrected are seen. Severe overcorrections are also possible. We have three cases that are as hyperopic now as they were myopic before surgery, including one −8 diopter myope who is now a +8.50 hyperope. Astigmatism, while helped in most cases, may show no improvement at all, and in some cases may be worse.

Patients are advised that the foggy, steamy vision which represents true glare rarely persists after one or two weeks of healing. It is seen only with small clear zones, excessive scarring, or cuts concentric with the pupillary margin. Radial cuts apparently produce a spoke wheel or star burst pattern with the rays equal in number to the number of radials the patient received in surgery. This star pattern appears only against a black background with pinpoint light sources. It does not block out road signs, street addresses, and other well-illuminated billboards at night. Some patients will have occasional night glare, principally if they are significantly undercorrected. The star pattern or flare is rarely found to impair night vision enough to force the patient not to drive. The star pattern fades considerably with time and can only be detected after a year with conscious effort on the part of the patient.

Patients are informed that fluctuating vision occurs because the corneal curvature varies during the waking hours. It is true whether the patient works nights or days. The most likely cause is dehydration of an overly hydrated cornea. In addition, steroids and diurnal pressure variation probably contribute to this phenomenon. Occasionally as much as one diopter can be noted between early morning readings and late evening readings. The keratometry readings confirm the refractive findings. A half-diopter is average, and in our cases, fluctuating vision has decreased with the passage of time. We have not seen a case that would require the fitting of two different pair of glasses except in normal presbyopia.

It is essential for the patient to realize that the effects of keratotomy appear to be permanent. "There is no eraser on the end of a diamond scalpel." There are few ways to reverse the effects of radial keratotomy surgery. While it is conceivable that further surgery may eliminate some cases of undercorrection, at the present time there are limited ways to undo an overcorrection. For that matter, a perfect correction cannot be undone in a case of a patient who later regrets the loss of the near vision which myopia afforded before presbyopia set in. The very permanence that is advantageous to a patient with an excellent emmetropic correction becomes a liability to those patients with an overcorrection, or, to those people who have second thoughts about their blurred near vision once past the age of fifty.

All radial keratotomy patients must be informed of the loss of accommodation that occurs with the normal aging process, regardless of radial keratotomy. Emphasis can be achieved by stating simply that *anyone* with 20/20 vision in both eyes will be completely unable to read a newspaper, telephone book, menu or price tag after the age of fifty; *only* people with residual *myopia* will be able to read without the aid of a reading device after that age. While reasonably intelligent patients can understand this fact intellectually, they do not understand the emotional impact of presbyopia. Therefore, they are unable to weigh this factor heavily enough in their risk/benefit equation until the following demonstration has been carried out: while under the effects of complete cycloplegia and with their full distant correction in place, the patient is asked to read fine print. Though they will say they understood the problem of presbyopia and its significance, they will nevertheless express amazement when this demonstration is carried out. It is particularly important and very effective to carry out this demonstration when discussing the advisability of doing surgery on the second eye after the first eye has achieved 20/20 vision. Many patients in the mild 1 to 3 diopter group will pause and take more time to consider their decision to have surgery on their second eye.

Patient Expectations. Many prospective radial keratotomy patients have unrealistically high expectations. They may read overly enthusiastic articles or reports or may chat with excessively exuberant patients. Some of these patients find that 20/40 vision is fantastic, while others may find 20/20 with slight distortion is unsatisfactory. A graphic means to help bring patient expectations in line with reality is to use a fogging technique. This can be accomplished in two ways: first, the patient's glasses are removed and lenses are held up approximating 50%, 75%, 90%, and 100% of their clinical correction. The various percentages of people achieving these results can then be described to the patient. Secondly, when screening larger numbers of patients, it is often easier to have +1, +2 and +3 lenses handy; then, by using these over the patient's clinical correction, various percentages of gain can be demonstrated. Thus, a 6 diopter myope with full correction in place can be fogged to 50% by simply holding up a +3. Switching to a +2 would show the patient what a 65% to 70% improvement would look like; finally, holding up a +1 would give them an idea of what an 85% correction would be like. It should blur them to approximately 20/60. Thus, if 85% to 90% of the people with that degree of myopia are achieving 20/40 vision, the patient can be told this is a reasonable expectation. It also can be emphasized that 10 to 15 out of 100 patients will have results no better than that.

The fogging technique is of minimal value in mild myopes, that is, from 1 to 3 diopters of myopia, since this group needs 20/40 or better to achieve any significant benefit from the surgery. In the moderate, and particularly in the severe group, a partial correction may be highly desirable to one patient and yet totally inadequate to another. Words do not convey this well. Therefore, the fogging technique is most helpful in achieving a realistic understanding of the capabilities of radial keratotomy to improve but not always to eliminate refractive errors.

As the surgeon's experience in radial keratotomy increases, he will find that many of his new patients know several of his former patients and have discussed the surgery with them. Obviously, a patient with this much background in radial keratotomy does not need as thorough an educational program as the patient who reads an article in the press and comes to the physician without any prior opportunity to discuss the surgery. In this situation, the physician may wish to instruct his office staff to begin a two-level patient education program in which those with little or no background in radial keratotomy would receive an extensive workshop. Those with much information about the process of work-up, surgery, and postoperative care would only require that the more important factors be emphasized. Their counseling includes the possible, but infrequent, complications and difficulties. This information is important since former patients with good results might not know about the infrequent problems and complications.

Second Eyes. Most patients assume that if they achieve a good result on the first eye, they will need to have the second eye done. Obviously, if the degree of myopia is mild and the unoperated eye has 2 diopters or less myopia, there is a distinct advantage in leaving the second eye unoperated to compensate for the problems of presbyopia. Similarly, patients who have a perfect 20/20 result in one eye, and only 20/100 as a result of surgery in their other eye, often ask whether the eye with the poorer vision should be reoperated. The advantage of leaving this eye undercorrected to compensate for presbyopia is a valid one. Some physicians are purposely undercorrecting one of the two eyes in order to achieve this highly desirable result. Approximately 80% of patients who have less than 2 diopters of anisometropia are able to achieve comfortable binocular vision and do not need any compensating device, or further surgery.

Occasionally night driving will be a problem, because of the undercorrected or myopic eye. A few patients will wear a spectacle correction as an option, though not as a necessity, to improve their night vision. Obviously, they must be allowed the opportunity of further surgery. However, it often seems that an optional pair of night driving glasses is more desirable than the absolute necessity of wearing reading correction for the last half of the person's life. Patients are not easily convinced of the practicality and advisability of refraining from surgery on the second eye, or of not repeating surgery on an undercorrected eye. Several points can be very useful in helping the patient recognize this advantage. One is to render the 20/20 postoperative eye cycloplegic and ask the patient to read fine print. They frequently are shocked as to just how blurred their near vision is, and readily agree that they need to think about the decision.

It is not always possible to achieve as perfect a correction in the second eye as has been done on the first eye. There are definite possibilities of under- and overcorrections, even though we attempt to do exactly the same surgery. It is also important to point out that the dangers of infection and distortion, which were true for the first eye, are factors in the consideration for surgery on the second eye. In many cases, the patient may be achieving reasonably good binocularity, even though one eye has not been operated on. Though patients may have some minor problems with diplopia, these problems may be considerably less than the nuisance and restriction that presbyopia will bring. Frequently the patient's instinct is to "even things up" and ask to go ahead with surgery. Again, this is the time to point out there is no way to undo the effects of radial keratotomy, and once operated upon, there is no way they can return to their myopic preoperative state.

Ophthalmologists should not be overly dogmatic and autocratic in these discussions since this may force patients to assume a defensive stance. This *is* counseling, and the decision is theirs and theirs alone; however, they must have the facts in order to make a decision they will not regret later on.

In some cases, the author has found it necessary to stress to the patient that, in counseling them not to do surgery on their second eye, we were actually turning away business. While the mention of the surgical fee may be somewhat crude, it may have a desirable effect on a patient who is not really listening, but is arguing and not thinking.

Since it takes several months for patients to become adapted to monovision, these discussions are best delayed until the three-month examination which is carried out under full cycloplegia. The patient who at one month postop was adamant that surgery would have to be done on the second eye is somewhat more hesitant by the second month and, by the third month is often willing to listen to reason. If this patient can be convinced that there is nothing to lose in waiting an additional few months, they often are quite comfortable by six months. Moreover, they almost never consider having surgery done on the second eye by the time they are one year postoperative. Thus, time is on the side of the position of settling for unilateral surgery. Naturally, there are exceptions to these rules. One must consider the needs of truck drivers, for example, especially those who drive at night; forklift operators; and perhaps most important of all, surgeons. While it must be pointed out to these individuals that reading glasses will become necessary, they invariably agree that is of secondary importance, and their primary need is to have good comfortable binocular vision now.

Interval Between Eyes. Since the risk of radial keratotomy appears to be quite low, the time between the first and second operation is arbitrary. Traditionally, three months was considered an adequate healing period in most eye operations. Therefore, our protocol was established requiring patients to wait three months between surgeries. This practice has been beneficial in a significant number of cases by allowing us to see how well the first eye did, and to give us time to tell that it apparently was stable. Many eyes achieve a stable endpoint before one month; however, others progress or regress during the ensuing 60 days, and what might have appeared to be an under- or overcorrection changes. Thus a more accurate surgical procedure can be done on the second eye by waiting the full 90 days between surgeries. Most patients hope never to require repeat surgery and it seems highly desirable to do everything which gives the patient the greatest chance of success. There are exceptions, and these need to be considered individually. In our experience no situation has arisen where there was harm or loss of a good correction by waiting three months or more. However, if a physician feels that stability has been achieved at an earlier stage and he wants to proceed with the second eye, this certainly is his decision.

Selection Factors

Psychological Factors. Many of the factors involved in patient counseling which were described in the preceding section can also be considered as selection screens. For instance, a patient with unrealistic expectations should be a sign that the physician needs to carefully recounsel the patient. He may find it necessary to reject patients if they do not have realistic expectations. A −9 diopter myope who will not be satisfied with anything less than 20/20 vision has less than a 1 in 10 chance of realizing his goal, and that patient certainly should be rejected for surgery. This is also true of the patient who is unable to understand the risks of the surgery or to understand that the surgery is not always exactly predictable. Some high myopes do not seem able to comprehend why they do not have as good a chance of achieving 20/20 as milder myopes do. If further counseling cannot make this clear to them, surgery should be avoided.

Physical Factors. The physical factors which serve as a basis for the selection of patients include: age, degree of myopia, degree of astigmatism, keratometry, corneal diameter, corneal thickness, tonometry, corneal shape, and visual acuity. Each of these factors will be discussed, and the normal range to be expected in the myopic patient population will be defined.

Age—Range: 18 to 60. Although the majority of keratorefractive surgeons feel that 18 is the minimum age for a person to be eligible for radial keratotomy, many are more comfortable operating only if the patients are 21 to 23 years of age or older for these reasons: 1) Young people do not achieve as much surgical correction with the same amount of surgery as older people do. While this can be compensated for by being more aggressive and using a smaller clear zone, the younger patient will have more glare, more fluctuation, and more distortion than the older patient. For instance, a 4 diopter myope normally will require a 3.5 to 3.75 mm clear zone, but a young patient will require a 3.0 mm clear zone. In contrast, an older patient past the age of 40 will not need a clear zone any smaller than 4.0 mm. 2) Psychologically, young people have less experience with life's trials. They are often not as realistic in their ability to grasp the risks and understand the nature of statistical averages. Thus, they are less able to realize that if 80% of the patients in their category get a 20/40 or better result, that means 20% get less than that and they must be psychologically prepared to deal with that shortcoming. 3) In most cases, a young patient has not had an ample opportunity to work with the various types of contact lenses. The older patient, however, may have tried several different kinds of lenses and no longer be successful with any of them. They are much more appreciative of the advantages that keratotomy has to offer and much more understanding of its shortcomings. 4) Younger people need to be concerned with the fact that their keratotomy is going to have to withstand the rigors of time in excess of 50 to 60 years. Since knowledge of the long-term effect is not available yet, they are taking a somewhat greater risk than the older patient.

Degree of Myopia—Range: −1 to −10 Diopters. In a sense, radial keratotomy can be thought of as three operations. By breaking the degree of myopia into three ranges, we are able to understand prospective patients better, because these three groups react in a somewhat different manner. The three groups are: −1 to −3 diopters (mild), −3 to −6 (moderate), and −6 to −10 (severe). Table 3-1 summarizes the expectations in these groups. In general, radial keratotomy is of limited benefit for people with over 10 diopters of myopia.

There appears to be little gain from a correction of only 50% in the mild group (-1 to -3 diopters of myopia). The patient who can already read without glasses and can see a reasonably sized clock at the bedside does not gain significant improvement unless 20/40 or better vision is achieved. Fortunately, 19 out of 20 are found to do this in a carefully controlled series, but that still leaves one person in twenty who does not. Each person must recognize that this possibility exists. Approximately 15% of our patients are in the mild group. This represents a small fraction of the adult myopic population, three-fourths of whom are "mild." This suggests that most mild myopes are not motivated enough to consider surgery an acceptable alternative.

The moderate group consists of patients with -3 to -6 diopters of myopia. They have a great deal of benefit to gain from radial keratotomy, and the predictability formula we use appears to be quite adequate in the majority of these cases. More than 90% of these patients can achieve 20/40 or better, and between 50% and 60% can achieve 20/20. Even a partial correction will enable them to see a clock at a bedside table much more clearly. After surgery almost all of them are able to read a book comfortably without the use of lenses at a normal reading distance. There appear to be few complications in this group. The extremely small clear zones with recutting and extremely deep cutting are not necessary, so irregular astigmatism, severe night glare, moderate fluctuation, and significant distortion are avoided. Approximately 60% of the patients seeking radial keratotomy are in this group. Even partial correction has significant benefits so if they are carefully screened, and are aware not everyone achieves 20/20, they are a very satisfied group.

The high group, -6 to -10 diopters of myopia, is highly motivated and the most eager to consider surgery. High myopes are completely helpless without a corrective lens and in dire emergencies may be unable to function. They cannot drive a car or run from danger. However, RK surgery is being pushed to its limits in many of these cases. The results are more capricious. Under corrections and even extreme overcorrections can occur. Irregular astigmatism is more pronounced. The extremely small clear zones, occasionally as small as 2.7 mm, result in more night glare and occasionally in some daytime glare. Since the depth of cut often exceeds 95% in order to achieve full correction, these patients may have progressive cell losses because of greater flexing of the cornea. Frequently, they have 16 rather than eight incisions and, because of the small clear zone, the radial incisions are of the greatest length, causing more extreme peripheral bulging and therefore more corrective central flattening. It is more difficult to fit contact lenses to these patients because of the greater change in corneal architecture. However, since the extreme changes in corneal architecture occur in those cases which have the greatest correction, there is usually no need to fit them with contact lenses. Conversely, cases with the greatest *under*correction have the most uniform and regular corneas; they can, as a rule, wear contact lenses if they were able to wear them preoperatively. Although only a very small percentage of the general population falls into the severe myopia group, they comprise 25% of the patients having radial keratotomy performed.

Degree of Astigmatism—Range: .25 to 4.0. Astigmatism is present in nearly all patients, and yet most have no concept of its effect on their vision. Although we can assure most patients with less than 1 diopter of astigmatism that it is of little consequence, occasionally a patient with only .50 or .75 diopters of astigmatism will have some reduction in uncorrected acuity and find the result is less than optimal. Moderate degrees of astigmatism from 1 to 2.5 diopters can be corrected with radial keratotomy, but the results are less predictable than are the results in cases of simple myopia. It is possible to achieve no improvement in the astigmatism at all and, in some cases, the astigmatism can be made worse.

While many patients with large degrees of astigmatism can be corrected, this is not always the case. Many of those who are very nearsighted; that is -7, -8, or -9 diopters, may have moderate cylinders of 2, 2.5, or 3 diopters and, even if the astigmatism is not improved at all, complete elimination of the myopia will result in a highly satisfied patient in most cases. However, it would be advantageous if at least half of the cylinder could be eliminated. Patient satisfaction would then be significantly increased. The most important factor is to inform the patient that astigmatism results are rather unpredictable and significant residual astigmatism may be present after surgery.

Visual Acuity—Best Corrected Vision: Normal Range of 20/15 to 20/40. The best corrected visual acuity in most patients will be 20/20 or better. It is necessary to make clear to any patients whose best corrected acuity is less than 20/20 that there is little reason to expect radial keratotomy to improve this level of vision. In less than 5% of the cases, some improved best corrected acuity is seen. Since most of these cases are in the high myopic range, they are balanced by an almost equal number who may lose a line of best corrected acuity. While radial keratotomy can be performed on patients whose best corrected acuity is less than 20/40, a very careful analysis of patients needs and expectations and the reason for doing this surgery must be undertaken.

The underlying reason for the patient's decreased vision is of great importance. If extreme myopia is resulting in a Fuch's spot, the patient should be considered for a sling procedure. If the reduction in acuity is due to macular disease, radial keratotomy obviously would not be beneficial. The presence of senile cataracts is a contraindication for radial keratotomy since the surgery for the cataract would render the effects of radial keratotomy completely pointless. For patients with amblyopia in one eye, radial keratotomy can reduce any myopic correction they might have, but there may be no gain in visual acuity.

Since radial keratotomy has not reached the point where surgery on a one-eyed patient is prudent or acceptable, only one case of amblyopia has been permitted to have surgery, and then *only* on the amblyopic eye. The -10 diopter right eye, with correctable vision to 20/20, was not permitted to have surgery. Since no diplopia occurred when the 20/50 amblyopic left eye was corrected with a -10 lens, surgery in this eye was permissible; it resulted in an uncorrected visual acuity of 20/60 which was correctable with a -1 diopter lens to 20/50. The gain for this patient was being able to function adequately and safely, without the use of corrective lenses.

Keratometry—Normal Range: 40.00 to 48.00. In our experience, no patient with keratometry readings below 40.00 diopters has undergone surgery. There would be no reason not to consider mild to moderate correction up to 5 diopters of myopia if such a patient did present. However, greater amounts than 5 diopters would necessitate corneal flattening to below 35 diopters and that seems to cause greater than average distortion, glare, and variability of vision. A slight increase in the amount of surgical correction is seen as keratometry readings increase. However, keratometry measurements of over 48 should alert the surgeon to possible keratoconus. There is some clinical evidence that patients with keratoconus will have progressive flattening, hyperopia, and scarring as a result of radial keratotomy surgery. Documentation is minimal, but caution is advised.

Corneal Diameter—Normal Range: 11 mm to 13 mm. The vast majority of patients presenting for surgery will have corneas approximately 12 mm in diameter. Corneas smaller than 11 mm do tend to give less correction, and a smaller clear zone is necessary. Significant reduction in corneal size should alert one to the possible existence of other congenital ocular defects which might rule out this patient for surgery. Corneal diameters of over 13 mm apparently enhance the correction of radial keratotomy. Therefore, to prevent significant hyperopia, it may be necessary to scale back the surgery by enlarging the clear zone.

Corneal Thickness—Normal Range: .47 to .64 mm. Most patients presenting for radial keratotomy will have corneal thickness between .52 and .56 mm. Accurate measurements of the cornea thickness centrally, paracentrally, and in the mid-periphery, are essential for correct blade setting. It has been suggested that corneas out of the range of normal may tend to undercorrect or overcorrect. Since it is possible that the pachymetry is not accurate, these judgments must be considered cautiously. Very thin corneas occasionally will be markedly inconsistent in thickness; therefore, careful corneal mapping is necessary to be sure to avoid perforation. Conversely, readings thicker than .60 mm may require careful blade setting in order to achieve adequate depth of incision.

Tonometry—Normal Range: 10 to 20 mm Hg. While an applanation tonometer is a very accurate tool, patient tenseness, slight pressure on the lid from the examiner's finger, and general lack of precision when taking pressures down in the lower normal range of under 16 mm Hg tend to obscure the fact that intraocular pressure has a significant bearing on the result of radial keratotomy. Patients with pressures below 10 mm Hg should be analyzed carefully, and the possibility of regular marijuana use must be considered; there is strongly suggestive anecdotal information that many undercorrections are the result of surgery on marijuana users. This type of smoking is prevalent in the age group considering radial keratotomy. Young patients, particularly female, who also have very low intraocular pressure, no matter what the cause, are poor candidates for large radial keratotomy corrections.

Surgery on patients with intraocular pressures above 20 mm Hg is associated with large changes in corneal curvature. It is necessary to reduce the aggressiveness of the surgery in order to prevent overcorrection. These patients do quite well if the appropriate surgery is done. They are representative of a group of extremely pleased patients, most of whom are in the 40 to 50 age group. They are almost incredulous of being able to function without glasses after all these years; most have long since given up any hope that this would ever be possible. However, no patient with poorly controlled glaucoma should be considered for the surgery, and patients with even borderline pressures must be approached with caution.

Ocular Dominance. Ocular dominance is particularly important in the mild group of myopes from 1 to 3 diopters since they frequently can achieve comfortable and high levels of ocular function with unilateral surgery. However, it must be surgery on the dominant eye. Determining which eye is dominant is not always easy. We use a card with a ¾" hole which the patient holds with *both* hands as he or she looks at the projected letter chart through a full distant correction, and then lifts the card to eye level. He moves it until he can see the 20/200 "E." If there is any doubt as to which eye the patient is using, he can be instructed to bring the card closer and closer to his eye. It will become obvious which eye he has chosen to use.

An additional test involves having the patient hold a finger 8" to 10" in front of his eyes, exactly in the midline between the two eyes, and then having him observe the "E" at the end of the room. The patient is then asked if he is aware of two ghost-like images of his finger in the foreground. He is cautioned not to look at these images, but to continue to look at the "E" and then note whether one of the ghost-like images is more solid appearing than the other. A more solid appearing left hand image means the right eye is dominant. This test more clearly defines which eye the patient suppresses, and which eye is dominant. The former test is more demonstrative of which eye the patient chooses to "aim with." Both tests are subject to error, and sometimes there appears to be very little dominance. Where little dominance exists, most patients prefer the right eye for distance since they back up the car by using the right eye as they look over their right shoulder. They tend to use a camera and most aim with their right eye. However, a truly left eye dominant patient should have surgery on that eye if he is in the mild 1-3 diopter group.

In myopes with greater than 4 diopters of myopia, where surgery almost certainly will have to be done on both eyes, the non-dominant, usually left eye, should be operated first. If the results are not optimal, the surgical parameters can be adjusted and the redesigned surgery can be performed on the dominant eye, giving this eye a better chance for 20/20 vision.

Summary

While the scientific basis for the efficacy of radial keratotomy may rest on the percentage of patients achieving 20/20 to 20/40 vision or having postoperative refraction within +1 to −1 diopter of emmetropia, the final analysis of the success of radial keratotomy depends on a satisfied and happy patient. Over-promotion of radial keratotomy as a means of eliminating a person's need for glasses or contact lenses can only result in a large percentage of dissatisfied patients whose expectations have not and could not have been met.

Radial keratotomy is a useful but imprecise tool. It can eliminate much of a patient's myopia and some astigmatism. However, until we can get 20/20 or better vision in 98% of the cases without serious residual hyperopia, it is important that the patient have a clear understanding of the capriciousness of the outcome. They might even be told that, in a sense, they are "reaching into a grab bag." It is of further importance they have some concept of the possibility of having glare, fluctuating vision, and ghost images postoperatively. While these minor complications do improve with time, they do not always go away completely; they may appear very minor to a patient with a good correction, but they can be quite significant to a patient who has achieved a suboptimal correction. Finally, patients must clearly understand the implications of progressive cell loss as well as the possibility of long-term complications and other problems which may occur late in the postoperative period. If properly forewarned of these effects, the vast majority of patients who proceed with surgery will find it is an extremely fulfilling and highly gratifying endeavor; moreover, they usually will express a great deal of gratitude to the physician who has helped them achieve it.

Chapter 4

Preoperative Evaluation

Robert F. Hofmann, MD

PREOPERATIVE EVALUATION

Radial keratotomy (RK) is a form of incisional refractive keratoplasty in which the goal is to accomplish emmetropia through the precise placement of consistent cornea-relaxing incisions. Within limits, the procedure is quite effective,[1-5] but as yet somewhat unpredictable. The two main sources of error are the present lack of standardization of surgical technique and the lack of precise delineation of surgical parameters.[1,5,6] The instrumentation currently available to evaluate the prospective RK surgery patient is that which is commonly available in the ophthalmologist's office. Few new instruments have been specifically developed to precisely determine the operative parameters necessary to predict the exact result in a particular patient. The two most important surgical parameters which should be derived in the RK patient are the size of the optical zone and the depth of the incision desired. Ideally, the entire structure of the cornea including the dimensions of the base of the dome, thickness at all points, surface curvature, and other data should be determined. Mathematical models such as those presented by Schachar,[7] are complex in their non-linear form and are difficult equations to solve even on sophisticated mainframe computers. On the other hand, the statistical programs currently available[1,8,9] utilize multivariant regression analysis to determine a best-fit nomogram. The statistical models do not assure absolute precision, but they are the best means currently available. The use of structural models is limited by the tools with which we measure the cornea, and the statistical models limit the surgeon because of the inherent variability of biological systems.

Essential Examination

Keratometry. Most current radial keratotomy nomograms require central keratometry values. Dioptric values of between 40.00 and 48.00 are the limits best advised for this surgery. Extremely flat corneas are difficult to flatten more than one to two diopters, because persistent postoperative values less than 37.00 are rarely achieved. Steep corneas, especially those with distorted mires, often develop anterior keratoconus, which does poorly in response to RK surgery. The condition of the reflex mires also indicates the regularity of the surface in long-term hard contact lens patients. Contact lens patients may require a period of two to eight weeks without wearing their lenses for stabilization of the refraction in the corneal surface prior to making any surgical decision.

As useful as the keratometer is, it has some distinct limitations for our purposes. The central curvature of the cornea as measured by the Bausch & Lomb keratometer (Figure 4-1) is an averaged reading[10] over a 3.5 mm zone (Figure 4-2). The standard diagnostic keratometers also are unable to precisely locate the visual axis or the structural apex of the cornea. The

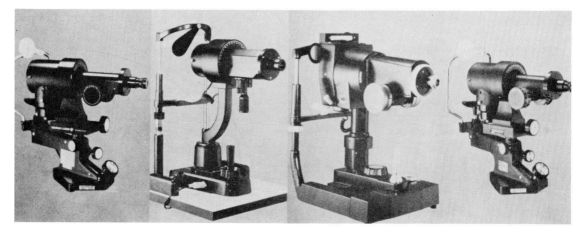

Figure 4-1. Standard keratometers clinically available in most offices can be used with current nomograms for radial keratotomy.

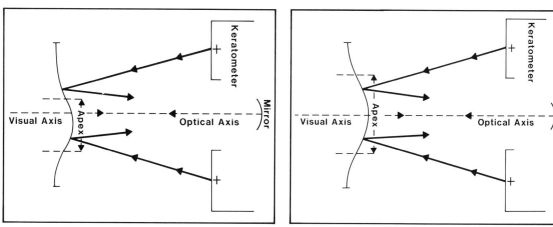

Figure 4-2A.

Figure 4-2B.

Figures 4-2A and B. Standard clinical keratometry averages radius of curvature over the central 4.0 mm of the cornea. Regardless of the size of the apex or the instantaneous changes within the central zone, this clinical averaging can yield the same keratometric readings. Figures 4-2A and 4-2B have the same keratometric readings despite different topography and apex size.

measurement attained in diopters is a derived value based upon an assumed index of refraction (n = 1.3375) of the human cornea. Nevertheless, until a more predictive means of relating total corneal topography to surgical results is presented, the Bausch & Lomb style keratometer remains the standard.

The automated keratometric devices[11] (Figure 4-3) can be more consistent than operator-manipulated standard keratometers. The automated devices make an attempt to determine a "shape factor" for the cornea, but no one has yet published detailed results relating so-called "shape factors" to the surgical outcome from radial keratotomy. The theoretically best means of assessing total curvature would be to measure the entire topography of the cornea and relate total, as well as instantaneous, surface changes to the desired effect from the keratotomy incisions. Yet, until recently, the means to digitize and interpret a precise, well-focused corneascope map in a facile and inexpensive manner has been lacking. The standard cor-

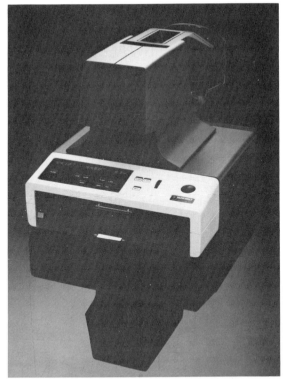

Figure 4-3A.

```
NAUTOKERATOMETER
        SEQ NO. 04
-----------------

RIGHT EYE

  CENTRAL K
   DK     mm   AXIS
   44.62  7.57 164
   45.62  7.39  74

  ΔK  -1.00DK ×164

  APICAL K
   DK     mm   AXIS
   44.75  7.54 162
   45.62  7.38  72

  ΔK   -.87DK ×162

  SHAPE    +.18
  APEX      .17 IN
            .08 DN
            .41TOL
  CONF.     92%
-----------------

LEFT EYE

  CENTRAL K
   DK     mm   AXIS
   44.12  7.64  11
   44.62  7.56 101

  ΔK   -.50DK × 11

  APICAL K
   DK     mm   AXIS
   44.12  7.65  17
   45.00  7.50 107

  ΔK   -.87DK × 17

  SHAPE    +.13
  APEX      .05 IN
            .15 UP
            .56TOL
  CONF.     83%
```

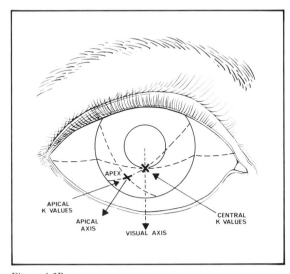

Figure 4-3B.

Figure 4-3C.

Figures 4-3A, B, and C. The Humphrey Automated Keratometer (A) is a computerized device for technician accumulation of keratometry data. (B) The Humphrey Keratometer analyzes the central curvature as well as paracentral curvatures of the cornea relating these readings to both the apical axis and the visual axis of the cornea. No direct correlation of this shape analysis to radial keratotomy has been defined despite the fact that radial keratotomy procedures alter the curvature of the central portion of the cornea about the visual axis which is generally nasal to the apical center of the cornea. (C) The printout for the Humphrey Keratometer lists central as well as paracentral keratometry relating the corneal shape about the visual axis and corneal apex. This printout is more useful in contact lens fitting than with radial keratotomy at present.

neascope[12,13] device is descriptive in its analysis but has not, as of yet, provided any predictive value to the radial keratotomy refractive surgeon. Perhaps with the development of the Kerascan Keratograph Auto-analyzer,[14] the equations regarding the shape of the cornea can be resolved so a computer may in the future actually determine the number and placement of the incisions to effect the desired outcome. The Kerascan Autoanalyzer (Figure 4-4) is a computer which provides digital interpretation (radius of curvature or dioptric power), of concentric ring reflexes in a rapid mode. Further research will be necessary to determine the application of these digitized points to the desired surgical result.

Refraction. The refraction should be carried out in both manifest and cycloplegic modes to attain proper standardization. The cycloplegic refraction determines the benchmark against which measurements pre- and postoperatively can be compared. The manifest refraction determines the everyday state of the patient's error, and this is the value which the surgeon seeks to modify. Both plus and minus cylinder refractions provide information useful to the surgeon, especially in astigmatic cases.[15] The minus cylinder form provides the myopic component for correction as well as the amount of the cylindrical component to be corrected by astigmatic procedures. Both the spherical and cylindrical component are to be considered separately, especially when the astigmatic incision has a relative steepening effect upon the meridian 90° to itself [Poisson's Ratio]. The details of these calculations are given in the chapter on astigmatism. The positive cylinder refraction form delineates the axis at which the steepest meridian is found, but this may or may not correspond to the steepest keratometric meridian. As is often seen, many astigmatic patients have a combination of lenticular as well as corneal astigmatism. If the surgeon were strictly to operate upon the corneal cylinder, the patient might be left with residual postoperative astigmatism.

The cycloplegic examination of refraction provides more than benchmark information. Placing the full distance correction in front of the cyclopleged eye can quite effectively demonstrate an expected late postoperative presbyopia. If the patient were to be asked to read in this state, the loss of near vision could be striking to the person whose career is dependent upon near vision. Many middle-aged myopic presbyopes have the misconception that RK surgery can alleviate the problems related to age and loss of accommodation. This demonstration can often prevent an undesirable outcome of ill-conceived surgery on the presbyope. It may also convince the −1.50 to −2.50 myopic presbyope of the wisdom of monocular surgery on the dominant eye.

Visual Acuity. After the determination of the refraction and curvature of the corneal dome, the visual acuity under best corrected circumstances is assessed. A standard Snellen projection or wall chart can be utilized; however, for research and study conditions, a Bailey-Lovie[16] Eye Chart from the National Eye Institute's "Early Treatment of Diabetic Retinopathy Study"[17,18] is more accurate. This chart is placed in a four-fluorescent-bulb box to be retro-illuminated against a room illumination of 100 foot candles. Auxiliary devices such as the Guyton-Minkowski Potential Acuity

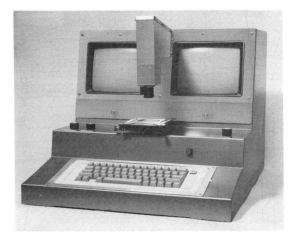

Figure 4-4A.

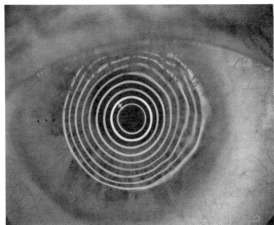

Figure 4-4B.

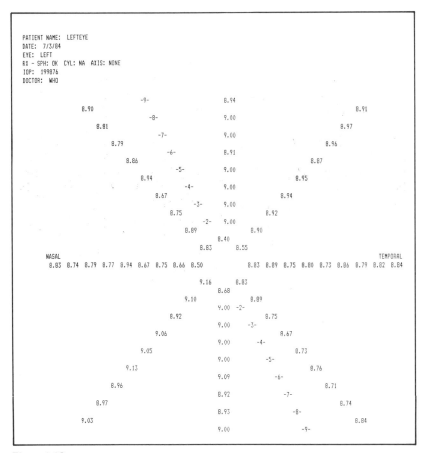

```
PATIENT NAME:  LEFTEYE
DATE:  7/3/84
EYE:  LEFT
RX - SPH: OK  CYL: NA  AXIS: NONE
IOP:  199876
DOCTOR:  WHO

                    -9-              8.94
         8.90                                          8.91
           8.81          -8-         9.00            8.97
                8.79     -7-         9.00          8.96
                    8.86  -6-        8.91
                          -5-        9.00        8.87
                    8.94             9.00       8.95
                          -4-        9.00
                    8.67             9.00      8.94
                          -3-        9.00
                     8.75            9.00     8.92
                          -2-        9.00
                      8.89           9.00  8.90
                               8.40
                          8.83    8.55
  NASAL                                                         TEMPORAL
  8.83 8.74 8.79 8.77 8.94 8.67 8.75 8.66 8.50   8.83 8.89 8.75 8.80 8.73 8.86 8.79 8.82 8.84

                          9.16     8.83
                               8.68
                     9.10            8.89
                          9.00  -2-
                    8.92             8.75
                          9.00  -3-
                9.06                8.67
                          9.00  -4-
             9.05                   8.73
                          9.00  -5-
          9.13                      8.76
                          9.09  -6-
        8.96                        8.71
                          8.92   -7-
     8.97                            8.74
                          8.93   -8-
   9.03                              8.84
                          9.00   -9-
```

Figure 4-4C.

Figures 4-4A, B, and C. The Kerascan Keratograph Autoanalyzer is a digital computer used to rapidly designate radius of curvature for 72 points on the corneascope photographic plate. Figure 4-4A shows the Kerascan microcomputer unit with interpreter. Figure 4-4B is a sample corneascope photographic plate. Figure 4-4C is a sample output from the digital interpretations of the photographic plate indicating instantaneous radius of curvature at each discrete point on the corneal topography.

Meter (PAM) can be useful in determining the actual macular acuity of the patient disregarding both minor opacities and refractive error. It is unsure whether the correction of severe astigmatism or anisometropia in an adult will yield a better postoperative result in an amblyopic eye than that predicted preoperatively. Such factors as stereo-acuity and color perception have also not been evaluated in the patient surgically corrected of his ametropia.

Corneal Structure. The structural parameters of the corneal dome can be measured for diameter, height, and rigidity. The pressure inside of the dome, as derived by applanation tonometry, can also be ascertained. However, one problem with each of these parameter determinations is that the current technology is not precise in determining the parameters that we desire. The measurement of corneal diameter using standard calipers has not been specified as to whether the measurements are based on a White-to-White, limbal, or internal Schwalbe's-to-Schwalbe's measurement. The size of the cornea varies horizontally, vertically, and in each diagonal measurement externally, and it may also vary by the same or a different degree internally. The internal measurements of the peripheral corneal base ring are extremely difficult to quantify. The derivation of internal corneal diameter cannot be derived from external approximations. Nevertheless, in mathematical and structural models of expansile shells,[19-21] it is the internal curvature as well as the support ring of the internal aspect of the dome which are the most important structures to be measured.

The measurement of the internal pressure beneath the corneal dome can be derived using Goldmann applanation tonometry. This measurement is a clinical approximation of the intraocular pressure because manometric measurement is clinically impossible in refractive keratoplasty due to its danger. The measurement of intraocular pressure without knowing the resilience and elasticity of the individual human cornea at individual points on the internal structure of the dome makes the mosaic of knowledge incomplete.[22-25] Attempts to measure the so-called scleral rigidity using Maklakov tonometry and Schiotz tonometry (Friedenwald Nomogram)[26] give an imprecise measurement of posterior globe resilience.[21] The inclusion of Maklakov tonometry data[27] (Figure 4-5) has not aided in prediction of radial keratotomy incisions. Perhaps the failing of these weighted surface resistance devices is due to the inability to give instantaneous readings at a discrete level necessary for the interpretation and engineering analysis of the cornea. The age of the patient has been used in various nomograms and rules of thumb but at present no cutoff times have been clearly elucidated. There still is considerable controversy between refractive keratoplasty investigators concerning the exact effect of age. Some authors, such as Thornton, have published guides which include a percentage increase in effect for those patients over 30 years of age. This "2%" rule is elucidated in the Thornton guide included in this text. Other authors, however, do not include any mention of age or sex in their nomograms.

Pachymetry. The corneal thickness in the paracentral, midperipheral, and peripheral locations is an important measurement from both a safety and efficacy standpoint. The corneal thickness can be determined by 1)

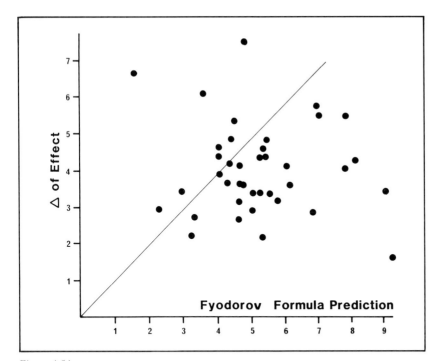

Figure 4-5A.

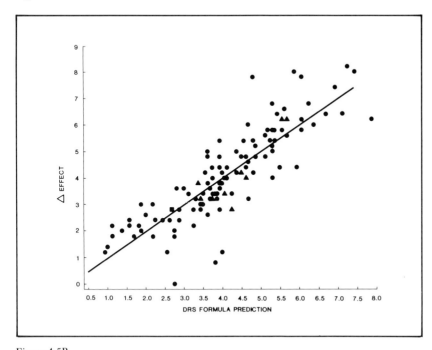

Figure 4-5B.

Figures 4-5A and B. Scatterplots demonstrating actual results vs. formula predictions. Figure 4-5A describes formula fit using original Fyodorov equations which require Maklakov tonometry. Oblique line indicates perfect fit. (Data from Hecht, SD, by permission). Figure 4-5B shows formula fit using Deitz, Retzlaff, Sanders (DRS) statistical formula with clinical manifestations. Circles = 1 patient; triangles = 2 patients; and squares = 3 patients. (Data from Deitz, MR, by permission).

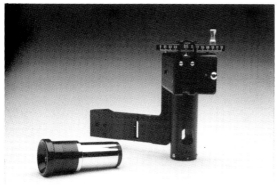

Figure 4-6A.

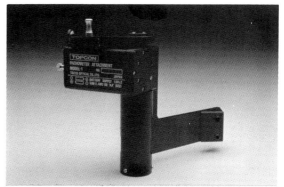

Figure 4-6B.

Figures 4-6A and B. Optical pachymetry using the Mishima-Hedbys fixation device is an inexpensive alternative to ultrasonic pachymetry and also has solved some of the alignment problems with standard Haag-Streit devices. Figure 4-6A shows the lighted scale, illumination slit, split mirror, and split image ocular. Figure 4-6B shows the double red alignment dots utilized to maintain perpendicularity of alignment with the corneal surface.

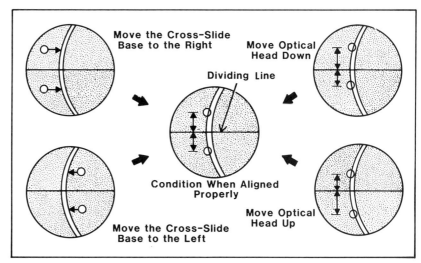

Figure 4-7. The alignment principle of the Mishima-Hedbys modification for the optical pachymeter utilizes two small red dots at 40° from the normal line from the corneal surface. When the red dots are aligned on the anterior surface of the epithelium equally separated onto the split beam image, alignment is significantly improved.

split beam optics, 2) interferometry, 3) electromechanical, and 4) ultrasonic means. All four techniques approach the determination of corneal thickness using certain assumptions, and it would be useful to know the inherent bias and benefit of each form.

With the addition of the Mishima-Hedbys' modification of the optical pachymeter[28] (Figures 4-6, 4-7), the problems with alignment were resolved for the paracentral horizontal and vertical measurements of the cornea. However, other problems with the optical pachymeter include difficulty in precise placement along the curvature, improper use by the surgeon, difficulty in diagonal quadrants and in the periphery, and non-use of correction tables by the surgeon. If the keratorefractive surgeon were to remember to use the brightest, thinnest beam with a precisely aligned slit to keep the epithelial image aligned along the red dots at a dioptric ocular correction of +2.00, then the optical method could provide a more precise end point than currently assumed. The surgeon should remember to measure from the anterior surface of the epithelium to the posterior surface of the endothelium using the split images. With the proper alignment of the slit image and an appropriate amount of practice, the optical device can be used in a facile and accurate manner. The surgeon must also correct his curvature readings using the correction tables supplied by the manufacturer (Figure 4-8). The optical pachymeter has a further advantage over the other types of thickness measuring devices in that it is inexpensive, atraumatic, and does not touch the cornea. The optical measuring device does not induce error by touching the structure upon which the measurements are taken.

Electromechanical devices (Figure 4-9) used in specular microscopes were originally designed for measuring the central and apical thickness of the cornea. These devices were not designed for use in refractive keratoplasty. Since the corneal thickness varies by quadrant as well as proximity to the center, the sole measurement of thickness in the center portion of the cornea using this type of device is inadequate. Another source of error in the electromechanical device is that the measurement derived is based upon the distance from the posterior surface of the tear film to the posterior surface of Descemet's membrane. The total corneal thickness, therefore, may be in error by as much as 20 to 30 microns. In the contact mode, the cornea is touched, compressed, and thereby modified, to give an abnormally thin reading. The inability to provide total corneal thickness in all diagonal points renders this mode of measuring inapplicable to refractive keratoplasty on a broad scale. The laser interferometric method[29] and the catoptric photographic method of Schachar[7] for measuring corneal thickness are not clinically available and are costly even for use in a research setting.

Ultrasonic pachymetry[30,31] (Figure 4-10) has undergone its first two generations of development over the past four years in the United States and Canada. The first units were somewhat difficult, variable, and subject to alignment error. The high cost of these instruments and the limited numbers of keratorefractive procedures done at that time also made the instruments of limited value. With the technological advances of alignment detection, storage and retrieval, mapping, sophisticated sampling algorithms, and decreasing probe tip size, these devices have been introduced both as presurgical and surgical evaluators of corneal thickness. The cost of the instrumentation also has been subjected to market pressures, thus decreasing the price significantly (Figures 4-11 and 4-12).

Prominent refractive surgeons have spoken highly of the advantages of ultrasonic pachymetry[30,31] but to date, no unbiased, independent laboratory evaluation of different brands of ultrasonic pachymeters has been reported. Various subjective impressions in a consumer's report format have been introduced at meetings but these, too, are also subject to observer bias. Perhaps the inability to match instrumentation is due to the fact that each machine has a different design philosophy. Some manufacturers believe that a solid probe tip is more precise at the probe/tear film interface while the proponents of the water-filled probe would say the same. These are all theoretical considerations which have not been subjected to rigorous scientific evaluation. The ultrasonic probe can be used both surgically and presurgically at random multiple points on the cornea with low inter-observer and inter-session variation. The opposite side of that argument is that the probe tip may be accurate at one particular location but it is difficult for the surgeon to precisely locate the same position using a hand-held probe under most clinical circumstances. No precise slit lamp or micro-scope-mounted device for accurate repeat placement and alignment of the

TOPCON
CORRECTING TABLE FOR PACHOMETER ATTACHMENT MODEL 1 FOR SL-3D

SCALE READING	CORNEAL RADIUS											
	5.5	6.0	6.5	7.0	7.5	8.0	8.5	9.0	9.5	10.0	10.5	11.0
0.04	0	0	0	0	0	0	0	0	0	0	0	0
0.08	0	0	0	0	0	0	0	0	0	0	0	0
0.12	−0.01	−0.01	−0.01	−0.01	−0.01	−0.01	0	0	0	0	0	0
0.16	−0.01	−0.01	−0.01	−0.01	−0.01	−0.01	−0.01	−0.01	−0.01	−0.01	−0.01	−0.01
0.20	−0.01	−0.01	−0.01	−0.01	−0.01	−0.01	−0.01	−0.01	−0.01	−0.01	−0.01	−0.01
0.24	−0.01	−0.01	−0.01	−0.01	−0.01	−0.01	−0.01	−0.01	−0.01	−0.01	−0.01	−0.01
0.28	−0.01	−0.01	−0.01	−0.01	−0.01	−0.01	−0.01	−0.01	−0.01	−0.01	−0.01	−0.01
0.32	−0.01	−0.01	−0.01	−0.01	−0.01	−0.01	−0.01	−0.01	−0.01	−0.01	−0.01	−0.01
0.36	−0.01	−0.01	−0.01	−0.01	−0.01	−0.01	−0.01	−0.01	−0.01	−0.01	−0.01	−0.01
0.40	−0.01	−0.01	−0.01	−0.01	−0.01	−0.01	−0.01	−0.01	−0.01	−0.01	−0.01	−0.01
0.44	−0.01	−0.01	−0.01	−0.01	−0.01	−0.01	−0.01	0	0	0	0	0
0.48	−0.01	−0.01	−0.01	0	0	0	0	0	0	0	0	0
0.52	−0.01	0	0	0	0	0	0	0	0	0	0.01	0.01
0.56	0	0	0	0	0.01	0.01	0.01	0.01	0.01	0.01	0.01	0.01
0.60	0	0	0.01	0.01	0.01	0.01	0.01	0.02	0.02	0.02	0.02	0.02
0.64	0.01	0.01	0.01	0.02	0.02	0.02	0.02	0.02	0.03	0.03	0.03	0.03
0.68	0.02	0.02	0.02	0.03	0.03	0.03	0.03	0.03	0.04	0.04	0.04	0.04
0.72	0.02	0.03	0.03	0.04	0.04	0.04	0.04	0.04	0.05	0.05	0.05	0.05
0.76	0.03	0.04	0.04	0.05	0.05	0.05	0.06	0.06	0.06	0.06	0.06	0.06
0.80	0.05	0.05	0.06	0.06	0.06	0.07	0.07	0.07	0.07	0.08	0.08	0.08
0.84	0.06	0.07	0.07	0.08	0.08	0.08	0.09	0.09	0.09	0.09	0.10	0.10
0.88	0.07	0.08	0.09	0.09	0.10	0.10	0.10	0.11	0.11	0.11	0.12	0.12
0.92	0.09	0.10	0.10	0.11	0.12	0.12	0.12	0.13	0.13	0.13	0.14	0.14
0.96	0.11	0.12	0.12	0.13	0.14	0.14	0.15	0.15	0.15	0.16	0.16	0.16
1.00	0.13	0.14	0.15	0.15	0.16	0.17	0.17	0.17	0.18	0.18	0.19	0.19
1.04	0.15	0.16	0.17	0.18	0.18	0.19	0.20	0.20	0.21	0.21	0.21	0.22
1.08	0.17	0.19	0.20	0.20	0.21	0.22	0.22	0.23	0.24	0.24	0.24	0.25
1.12	0.20	0.21	0.22	0.23	0.24	0.25	0.26	0.26	0.27	0.27	0.28	0.28
1.16	0.23	0.24	0.25	0.26	0.27	0.28	0.29	0.29	0.30	0.31	0.31	0.32
1.20	0.26	0.27	0.28	0.29	0.30	0.31	0.32	0.33	0.34	0.34	0.35	0.35

Real value = Scale reading + Correction
The table is based on refractive index of cornea of 1.376

Figure 4-8. The optical pachymetry method requires a correction table for the radius of curvature at each point. Without using the correction table, the thickness of the cornea as measured could be inaccurate by as much as ± 20 microns.

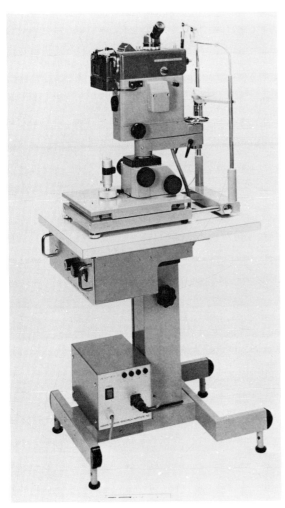

Figure 4-9A.

Figures 4-9A and B. Pachymetry by specular microscopy utilizes an electromechanical system for determination of corneal thickness through the camera system. This method of pachymetry is excellent only in the most central regions of the cornea. Alignment of the system in the paracentral and peripheral areas is difficult to attain. Figure 4-9A shows the complete view of the Pocklington specular microscope. Figure 4-9B details the digital electromechanical pachymetric system. The PRO Koester specular microscope also utilizes a similar system for corneal pachymetry.

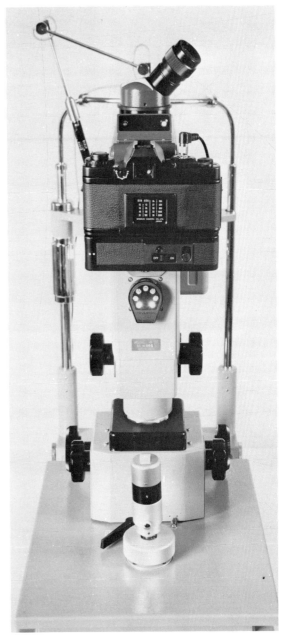

Figure 4-9B.

probe yet exists. When repeat measurements are taken, the surgeon is uncertain as to the exact alignment and placement of his probe for a second or third reading in the same location.

The fact that the ultrasonic probe touches the cornea means that the cornea has been altered. Solid probe units assume that the total corneal thickness starts at the anterior surface of the tear film and ends at the posterior surface of the endothelium. Fluid-filled devices measure from the anterior surface of the epithelium to the posterior surface of the endothelium. This variation in measuring may also be the reason some surgeons include "fudge factors" in their determination of the blade setting. The measurement of sound in the cornea has been variously assumed to be between 1620 and 1650 meters per second, and each manufacturer either standardizes to an assumed value or allows the surgeon to set his equipment to a preferred value. Various bias measurements can be programmed into the ultrasonic pachymeters based upon the surgeon's "clinical judgment," but this also lends to variability.

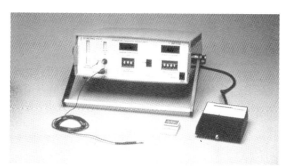

Figure 4-10A.

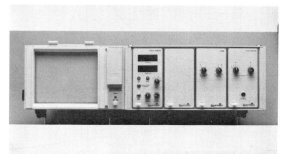

Figure 4-10B.

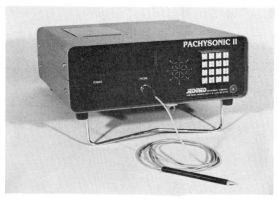

Figure 4-10C.

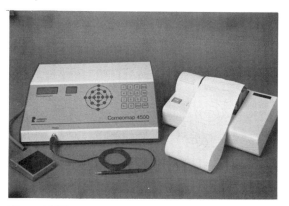

Figure 4-10D.

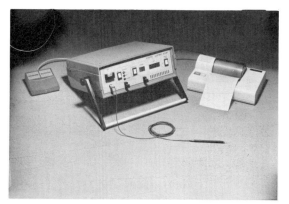

Figure 4-10E.

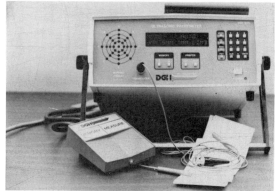

Figure 4-10F.

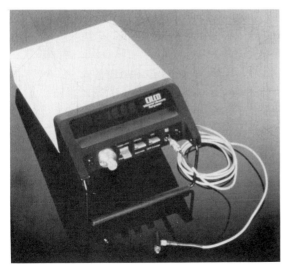

Figure 4-10G.
Figure 4-10. Commercially available ultrasonic pachymeters:
A) Accutome; B) CooperVision; C) JEDMED; D) Radionics;
E) Storz; F) DGH; G) CILCO.

The measurement of between 20 and 30 points on the corneal dome using ultrasonic pachymetry can be time consuming preoperatively even though with new surgical devices and templates, the knowledge may be essential in the future. Only the most motivated and stoic of patients can lie still for very long. Therefore, it is recommended that a limited number of points be measured using ultrasonic pachymetry at the paracentral and central zones as well as midperipheral zones in each of the diagonal quadrants. In most cases, the inferotemporal diagonal quadrant measurement tends to be the thinnest of any of the quadrants of the cornea and the most likely site for microperforation. The thinnest paracentral region multiplied by the bias factor of between 90% and 98%, depending upon the surgeon's plan, is selected for the initial incision. If the surgeon is planning to redeepen in the secondary or tertiary zone, then peripheral readings are taken. Mapping can be accomplished using the built-in printer with the unit or using a graphic plot supplied by the manufacturer or designed by the surgeon. Nevertheless, some care must be taken in planning the timing of the examination.

This author prefers to do pachymetry within 24 hours of surgery. At least a one week rest period from contact lenses should be imposed on the patient so that the cornea will be at its normal state of thickness. By performing pachymetry preoperatively, the examination can be done at leisure in the office without having the stress of surgery. If the probes are used intraoperatively to determine any measurements except paracentral readings, the cornea will be dried out enough to render an inaccurately thin reading of the cornea. The epithelium will also slough intraoperatively if exposed to topical anesthetics for a prolonged period. Whether mapped preoperatively or intraoperatively, the inability to page rapidly through the memory registers of the current class of pachymeters tends to slow measurement, which can be critical during surgery. Although at any one reading

Optical vs. Ultrasonic Pachymetry

	Optical	Ultrasonic
1. Number of Operators	One	One or More ·
2. Typical User	M.D. Only	M.D. or Technician
3. Training Required	Significant Experience Required for Consistency.	Less Than One Hour
4. Cost	Less Than $1000	Greater Than $5000
5. Observer Bias	Easy to be Subjective in Interpretation.	Not Completely Objective: Operator and Algorithm Bias Still Present.
6. Inter-Observer Bias	a) Left Eyes Read Thicker Than Right Eyes Due to Parallax. b) Different Observers Use Different End Points.	Low if Same Location Pinpointed and Corneal Hydration Consistent
7. Perpendicularity	Mishima-Hedbys Red Pinpoint Lights (Topcon)	Signal Sensors in Unit Won't Accept Echoes Unless Probe is Within 10 Degrees of Perpendicular to Surface.
8. Alter the Cornea or Tear Film	Non-Contact: No	SOLID HEAD PROBES: Yes FLUID PROBES: No, if Touch is Very Light.

Figure 4-11. Optical vs. Ultrasonic Pachymetry: Merit and Pitfalls.

in one location in a benchmark test the ultrasonic pachymeter is more accurate than the optical pachymeter, the total mapping of the cornea is somewhat more difficult using ultrasonic pachymetry. Perhaps a second or third generation of pachymeters, using other modalities (interferometry, holography, etc.) or advanced mapping, delivery and alignment devices

(cont'd)	Optical	Ultrasonic
9. Time to Map 9 Points	3 Minutes (approx.)	4 Minutes (approx.)
10. Accuracy	+/- 10 microns	+/- 5 microns
11. Ease to Patient	Comfortable at Slit Lamp	Usually Prone and Apprehensive About the Probe but Gives Good Assessment of Potential Behavior of Patient at Surgery.
12. Mounting	Slit Lamp Only	Free Hand or Some Slit Mounts
13. Use in Periphery	Fair to Poor	Good
14. Intraoperative Usage	None	Both Pre- or Intraoperative Intraoperative Failure of Instrument Cancels Surgery Unless Backup is Available. (Very Expensive)
15. Maintenace	Minimal - a Few Batteries for Pin Lites.	Unknown but Potentially Expensive for Repair and "Down" Time Loss of Surgical Revenue.
16. Improvements Expected	Laser Interfero-metric Devices in Development	Improved Mapping Registers, Fixation Diodes, Sampling Algorithms, and Probe Mounting. Costs will Decrease Due to Market Pressure.

could solve some of the problems inherent in early generation devices.

Despite the theoretical and practical limits of each modality, the refractive surgeon should settle upon one method. The weight of evidence indicates that most refractive surgeons can benefit from using ultrasonic pachymetry. The brand chosen is left to the discretion of the surgeon, as

Pachymeter Study   Spencer P. Thornton, M.D., F.A.C.S.

A

	Corneomap 4500 Radionics Medical Inc.	Kremer II Corneometer	Cilco 55 Villasenor	Coopervision	Jedmed Pachysonic II	Storz CS 1000	DGH 1000
One Operator	9	9	4	4	9	9	10
Reproduc-ability	10	10	2	5	7	10	10
Ease of Operation	7	7	8	5	8	6	9
Surgical & Postop Verification	10	10	4	NR	6	10	10
Mainten-ance Record	NR	8	6	NR	NR	NR	NR
Confidence Level	10	10	4	7	8	9	10
Portability	2	4	10	1	6	4	8

Scale 1-10 with 1=Poor 5=Average, 10=Excellent, NR=Not Rated (Too Little Experience)

Figure 4-12A.

B

	Corneomap 4500 Radionics Medical Inc.	Kremer II Corneometer	Cilco 55 Villasenor	Coopervision	Jedmed Pachysonic II	Storz CS 1000	DGH 1000
Price (Approx.)	$6500	$8500	$6000	$4500 Plus A&B Scan Unit	$5200	$5000 ($4350 s printer)	$6500
Weight	20lb.	10lb.	4lb.	45lb.	8lb.	10lb.	8lb.
Probe Tip Size	1mm	1mm	4.2mm	1.6mm	2mm	1.1mm	1.5mm
Probe Tip Type	Water	Water	Solid	Water	Solid	Water	Solid
Measurement Method	Pulse-Locked	Pulse-Locked	Average	Average	Average	Average	Average
Alignment Signal	Yes	Yes	No	No	Yes	Yes	Yes
Transducer	20 MHZ	20 MHZ	20 MHZ	20 MHZ	20 MHZ	20 MHZ	20 MHZ
Battery Compatible	No	No	Yes	No	No	Yes	No
Printer	Yes	Yes	No	No	Yes	Yes (Optional)	Yes
Instrument Accuracy	5µ	5µ	10µ	10µ	5µ	5µ	5µ

Figure 4-12B.

Figures 4-12A and B. Consumer ratings of ultrasonic pachymeters (by permission of Spencer P. Thornton, M.D.) compare the accuracy and other characteristics of currently available machines.

most of the units are quite accurate. Both surgeon and technician can obtain reliable results with ultrasonic pachymetry, and clinical evidence indicates a lower rate of surgical microperforation with it. The surgeon should frequently test the calibration of his instrument based upon a test block supplied by the manufacturer. His mapping sequence should be consistent and the surgeon must know the inherent bias of his machine prior to calculating the percent blade depth. As with any technique, ultrasonic pachymetry should be practiced so that eventually the reading can be confidently relied upon. Surgical depth cannot be ascertained by free-hand dissection or post-incision depth gauges, so the surgeon must trust his pachymeter implicitly.

Auxiliary Evaluation

Refractive incisional keratoplasty may be an investigational procedure in some form for a number of years yet. Just as the parameters defining the essential measurements necessary for the surgery have been discussed, the non-essential parameters will continue to be evaluated as they affect the patient's perception of his world. Those measurements used to evaluate the patient's subjective perception of his world preoperatively and postoperatively will have great bearing upon the long term acceptance of this procedure by the public.

Complete Eye Examination. The complete ophthalmic examination is essential in the evaluation of any eye surgical patient. Refractive keratoplasty structurally involves only the curvature of the anterior surface of the eye, but it has effects which weigh upon the entire visual system. From a medicolegal standpoint, the non-recognition of corneal, lenticular, posterior segment, and neuro-ophthalmologic pathology may lead to severe consequences. A thorough documentation of anterior and posterior segment pathology is essential for the protection of both the patient and the surgeon. Unless the patient knows of some structural or neurological limitation to best acuity postoperatively, he will not accept excuses when the postoperative result is not optimal. In patients who are highly myopic, macular and peripheral retinal pathology frequently can be found with a complete dilated examination. Photographic documentation of the anterior segment and fundus, although not essential, provides documentation which may be necessary later in the event of untoward medicolegal involvement. Since many myopes have peripheral retinal pathology, a complete dilated examination affords the surgeon the best opportunity to treat breaks or holes which were unrecognized prior to making radial or other cuts into the cornea.

Biometry. Axial biometry is commonly used in lens extraction, intra-ocular lens implantations, cryolathing refractive keratoplasty, and penetrating keratoplasty for the determination of probable postoperative refractive error. The ultrasonic biometer has been used quite accurately to measure the axial position. In incisional refractive keratoplasty, the A-scan length is immaterial to preoperative planning; in both laboratory and clinical models it has been shown not to vary significantly.[39,40] The slight variations noted in axial length are well within the error limits of the biometric probe. The anterior chamber depth for radial keratotomy has not been standardized because the exact location of the base of the corneal dome has yet to be determined. Optical means using the Haag-Streit attachment II are subject to the same inaccuracies of optical corneal pachymetry. No place for anterior chamber depth measurement has been indicated in any of the existing mathematical models. Since these measurements either do not vary or are within tolerable limits, and since they involve significant extra expense to the patient, they are not currently recommended in the routine workup of radial keratotomy patients.

Ocular Dominance. Ocular dominance is measured by the method of Scobee. Using a white piece of cardboard with a central hole of 2.5 cm diameter, the patient sights a Snellen letter at 20 feet with both eyes open. The patient then brings the cardboard toward the face rapidly and the hole ends up in front of the dominant eye. Subjective inquiries about handedness, "shooting eye," or camera fixating eye are inaccurate. In patients considering radial keratotomy or its variations, the question always arises as to which eye to operate upon first. In eyes that are relatively close in refractive error, the option has generally been to operate upon the nondominant eye first. The rationale for choosing the nondominant eye first is that the patient will be less affected by the aniseikonia and probable distortion of the fusional horopter. If complications were to occur, then the patient's preferred dominant eye would be unaffected if the patient chose not to have surgery on the second eye. However, in pairs of eyes which have significant anisometropia, the eye with the most myopic refractive error, even if it is the dominant eye, could be operated upon first. If that is the eye which most troubles the patient, the resolution of that myopia would set the outer limits of surgical technique and also give an indication as to the performance of that patient's cornea under surgical conditions. In either case, surgery on the second eye should be delayed until the first eye has been stabilized from a visual acuity and structural standpoint. This period of stability varies between three weeks and six weeks in most patients. Simultaneous operation upon both eyes may provide convenience to the

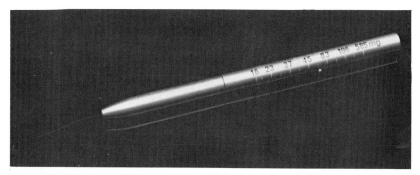

Figure 4-13. The Rowan Calibrated Corneal Aesthesiometer was developed by NASA and is an accurate device for assessing corneal sensitivity in an atraumatic manner.

surgeon but does not allow for the exact determination of postoperative result in the first eye in the calculations for surgery upon the second eye.

Near Point of Accommodation.
Most patients who are generally affluent and motivated enough to undergo radial keratotomy are those in their late 30's to early 40's. Frequently these patients have had multiple and unsuccessful attempts with contact lenses. With aging, the contact lenses can become uncomfortable due to tear film abnormalities. The fact that stress is placed upon upwardly mobile young executives to perform in an uncorrected ametropic world is not to be taken lightly. In these patients, the near point of accommodation must be measured, and the patient has to be counseled that presbyopia is inescapable as he ages.

Corneal Sensitivity.
Radial keratotomy and its astigmatic analogues involve cutting corneal nerves as well as collagen fibers. Sensitivity profiles, long- or short-term, do not exist for these procedures. The effect of various numbers and orientations of incisions upon corneal sensitivity has not been published. With the danger of post-RK herpetic keratitis documented, the hypesthesia of one eye in the pair with faint stromal opacification could signal significant risk. Hypesthesia could be noted in a high myope with previous 360° scleral buckle. The prolonged effects of a hypesthesia postoperatively are as yet undetermined. Data collection for corneal sensitivity is simple, inexpensive, and standardized. The Rowan Corneal Aesthesiometer (Figure 4-13) is a device containing a thin plastic filament of known diameter and length. The National Aeronautics and Space Administration (NASA) has calibrated the tension of the filament in milligrams for each length. The principle of the test is to successively shorten the filament until the patient responds verbally. Simple blinking or touch to the lashes leads to false positive results. Extensive instructions for the use of the Rowan Corneal Aesthesiometer are included with the instrument.

Glare Sensitivity Testing.
In approximately 20% of patients[32] who have undergone standard eight-incision radial keratotomy, glare is bothersome for the first three months postoperatively but is generally not a persistent problem after six months. Glare sensitivity is usually assessed by asking patients to evaluate their glare problem in subjective terms. However, a simple test using a pen-light lacks sufficient quantification as to the light scattering which tends to disperse off-center light over the retinal image, thus decreasing contrast. Light scattering can occur in radial keratotomy due to the incisions themselves or the peri-incisional edema. Generally, the glare sensitivity decreases significantly within a few weeks[2,5] but in procedures in which there are more than eight incisions, the sensitivity can persist over many months or years.[1]

Recently, a quantifiable measure of threshold glare sensitivity, the Miller-Nadler Glare Tester[33,34] was developed to assess contrast glare sensitivity thresholds. The Miller-Nadler Tester (Figure 4-14) is an inexpensive device which involves the use of 35 mm slide mounts in a self-contained slide projector. The glare device utilizes a Kodak Ektagraphic Audioviewer [Model 260] with a series of 24 specially prepared 35 mm slides. The center of each slide has a 40 mm circle containing a dark

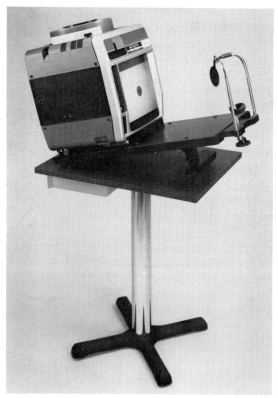

Figure 4-14. The Miller-Nadler Glare Tester (Titmus) is a clinical device used for assessment of light scattering from opacities in the ocular media as well as in the corneal architecture.

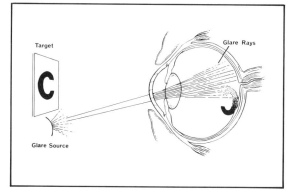

Figure 4-15. The glare testing system uses the principle of extraneous light scattering across the corneal incisions to wash out the retinal image of a central test object.

Landolt ring against a background of varying illumination (Figure 4-15). Surrounding the target is a large bright area representing the circular glare source of 2000 foot-Lamberts. The contrast levels within the series vary from 1% to 94%. A contrast of 94% means a dark ring against a light background whereas a slide of 1% contrast means a background almost as dark as the Landolt ring. At a testing distance of 36 cm, the target subtends an angle of 1° at 0.3 meters, producing the equivalent of a 20/200 Snellen letter. During the study, the endpoint or threshold is recorded as the last properly identified slide.

Glare sensitivity is variable even in the unoperated patient. Patients who tend to have high refractive errors, tear deficiencies, blue irides, high age, significantly high cylinder, and corneal or lens opacities may have a greater than normal glare sensitivity. The radial keratotomy patient has radial and transverse astigmatic incisions which involve a zone of 3.0 mm about the central visual axis to the periphery and the pupil can naturally dilate from a 2.5 mm zone to a 7.0 mm zone; therefore, there is significant chance for long-lasting glare with this procedure. Since the patient frequently complains of nighttime glare due to dark dilatation, night driving may be difficult for weeks and months after RK surgery. Transverse as well as trapezoidal Ruiz incisions near the visual axis would be expected to cause more glare and distortion than the simple thin linear incisions of a diamond-blade radial keratotomy. The introduction of thin incision diamond blades and the technique of going from center to periphery reduces the scar size and the damage to the epithelium and Bowman's membrane in the para-central zone.[35] The baseline appraisal of glare sensitivity, although not predictive for surgical purposes, is very instructional to the patients about to undergo refractive keratoplasty. The patient should be informed that, for the most part, persistent and severe glare tends to be transient in uncompli-cated radial keratotomy.

Psychometric Testing. The patient's expectations preoperatively and probable satisfaction postoperatively are difficult to assess in the clinical situation. There are innumerable reasons for a patient to seek refractive surgery. Not all reasons expressed by patients would seem on the surface to be valid to the ophthalmic surgeon who may or may not have a significant myopic refractive error. Transient flaws or expected side effects in an unstable patient may cause significant grief during the postoperative period.[36] Formal psychological testing is not generally applicable in the

---

Radial Keratotomy Patient Survey

The Ophthalmology Department is conducting a survey of all radial keratotomy patients at one year after their surgery. It is extremely important to us that you take a few minutes to respond so that we can better evaluate our results. We need your personal input and will be grateful for your cooperation. Please keep in mind that people who have elective surgery want to speak as positively about their results as possible and answer in as much detail as you wish.

1. Are you happy with the results of your surgery?

2. Do you have any reservations or disappointments about the surgery?

3. Before surgery, were you adequately informed about risks and complications?

4. Do you experience ANY increased glare?

5. Do you have increased difficulty driving at night?

6. Are there any new problems with your vision since your surgery?

7. Are you able to see satisfactorily without glasses?

8. What advice would you give a prospective radial keratotomy patient?

9. Has the quality of your life been changed by this surgery.

Figure 4-16. A sample patient survey for radial keratotomy can be devised by the individual practitioner to assess the patient's subjective perception of surgery performed previously. The feedback from such a system could benefit the surgeon greatly in assessing the benefits and risks of the surgery from the patient's viewpoint.

REFRACTIVE KERATOPLASTY STUDY PATIENT EXAMINATION SCHEDULE

	PRE-OP	1 DAY & 3 DAY	1 WK & 2 WK	1 MO	2 MOS	3 MOS	6 MOS	1 YR	2 YR +
Complete Eye Examination	X							X	X
Visual Acuity c & s R$_x$	X	X	X	X	X	X	X	X	X
Slit Lamp Examination	X	X	X	X	X	X	X	X	X
Manifest Refraction	X	X	X	X	X	X	X	X	X
Cycloplegic Refraction	X							X	X
Keratometry (by M.D.)	X	X	X	X	X	X	X	X	X
Photoelectric Keratometry	X							X	X
Applanation Tonometry	X		X	X	X	X	X	X	X
Pachymetry	X							X	X
Corneal Diameter	X							X	X
Corneal Sensitivity	X							X	X
Ultrasonography, Axial Length	X							X	X
Slit Lamp Photography	X							X	X
Specular Photographs	X							X	X
Anterior Chamber Depth (PSC — ASL)	X							X	X
Glare Testing	X							X	X
Potential Acuity (PAM)	X							X	X

CHECKLIST FOR REFRACTIVE KERATOPLASTY STUDY PATIENTS

INITIAL

	1	Complete Eye Examination
	2	Fulfills The Criteria For The Study
	3	Procedure and Investigative Study Explained
	4	Consent Explained and Signed
	5	Special Studies Completed and Report Filed
	6	Surgery Scheduled
	7	Surgery Performed 1st Eye and Report Filed
	8	Followup Visits Scheduled - First Eye R/L
	9	Surgery Performed 2nd Eye and Report Filed
	10	Followup Visits Scheduled - Second Eye R/L
	11	Followup Visits, Special Studies and Report Filed - 6 months
	12	One-Year Followup Completed and Report Filed
	13	Two-Year Followup Completed and Report Filed
	14	Three-Year Followup Completed and Report Filed
	15	Four-Year Followup Completed and Report Filed
	16	Five-Year Followup Completed and Report Filed

VISUAL ACUITY EQUIVALENTS

Snellen	20/15	20/20	20/25	20/30	20/40	20/50	20/60	20/70	20/80	20/100	20/200	20/400	10/400	5/400
Decimal	1.33	1.00	0.80	0.66	0.50	0.40	0.33	0.28	0.25	0.20	0.10	0.05	0.02	0.01

Figure 4-17A.

Figures 4-17A, B, C, D, and E. A) Protocol and schedule of examinations; B) baseline and annual examination form; C) diagrams for recording pachymetry and corneoscopy; D) surgical data form; E) postoperative minor visit form. Ongoing clinical research for refractive surgery is essential. The meticulous and accurate recording of results will go a long way toward improving the procedure's accuracy for future patients. Until a working structural model can be used to predict radial keratotomy, only by accurate regression analysis can the surgeon further refine his predictability.

average clinician's office, but the patient-physician relationship that is established during these first interviews can go a long way toward determining the patient's true candidacy at a psychological level for refractive keratoplasty. In the Prospective Evaluation of Radial Keratometry (PERK) study,[37,38,43] a psychometrist developed a psychometric test battery which contained standard questions from other widely used tests including the Rand Health Insurance Study, the Beck Depression Inventory and the Ware Patient Satisfaction Test as well as a series of questions designed specifically for use with radial keratotomy patients. The test was developed in the field using 100 radial keratotomy patients before it was revised and employed in the PERK study. The formal study measured factors such as demography and personality characteristics in those patients electing surgery as well as the source from which the patients learned about radial keratotomy. The patient's reasons for having radial keratotomy were assessed as were postoperative satisfaction. The final correlation between preoperative motivation, self-concept, and the amount of knowledge about the procedure with preoperative satisfaction and self-concept[38,43] were assessed in the study.

The data collected from the PERK study patients as compared to the Rand Health Insurance Experiment described the typical PERK radial keratotomy patient as being an affluent young white myope who has both a dislike for being dependent upon corrective lenses and also a fear of being without vision when the prosthesis is nonfunctional or missing. Most patients had previously tried contact lenses and had quit wearing them mainly because the use of the lenses was inconvenient or bothersome. There was no evidence in the study that the patients were psychologically or socially deviant. There also was no evidence that the patients sought radial keratotomy surgery for cosmetic or significant occupational reasons. The first of two primary motivating drives for the radial keratotomy patients is a true fear of being unable to see due to dependence upon ocular prosthetic devices. The patients were worried about what would happen if the eye glasses or contact lenses were lost in an emergency. The second motivating aspect which is highly inter-related with the first is a dislike of lenses with a sensation of inconvenience of any type of corrective lens.

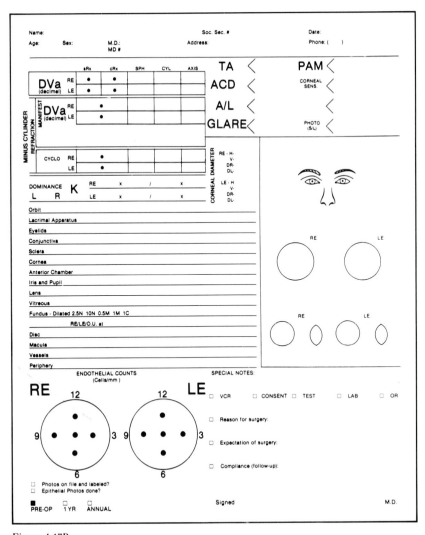

Figure 4-17B.

Such complaints as the spectacles distorting vision, facial discomfort, maintenance problems, and repeated costs were those complaints most commonly voiced by the PERK study patients. There was no way to distinguish clearly between feelings of general inconvenience and feelings of fear as motivations for surgery. Basically, the PERK study patients were active upper middle class affluent younger whites who perceived themselves to be more visually disabled than other myopes. They also disliked being dependent upon lenses of any type. Fear of being without vision and impatience with lenses motivate both males and females to seek this corrective surgery.[43]

This type of formal study is not feasible on a large scale in the average clinician's office but yet a modified questionnaire could be designed by the surgeon for interviewing the patient preoperatively in the form of a test associated with the videotape recording. Postoperatively an informal questionnaire (Figure 4-16) at six months, 12 months and 24 months could be

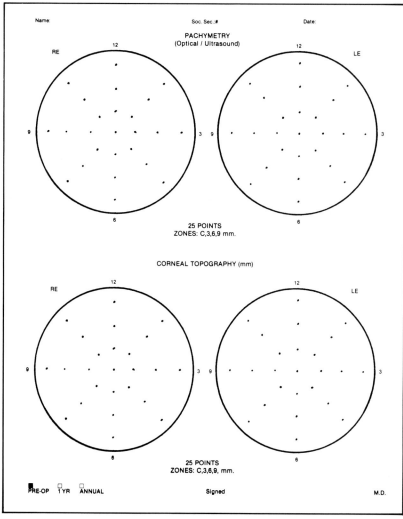

Figure 4-17C.

used. The results from this questionnaire would best be analyzed by an independent third source after the patient had completed the questionnaire in complete privacy.

Endothelial Specular Microscopy. The damage to endothelial cells from uncomplicated radial keratotomy is variable. The damage at the time of surgery has been variously assessed between 0%[1] and 10%[4] with an ongoing cell loss of 0% to 3%. The average cell loss in the laboratory and clinical situations from reoperations seems to be approximately 7%.[39,40] There has not been hard evidence in clinical studies of continuing significant endothelial cell loss or alteration in endothelial fluorescein permeability.[41] Original studies of endothelial cell density were flawed due to the fact that they measured only central or paracentral cellular density and because postoperative counts were performed by different technicians without precise methods of standardization. A fixation device, originally

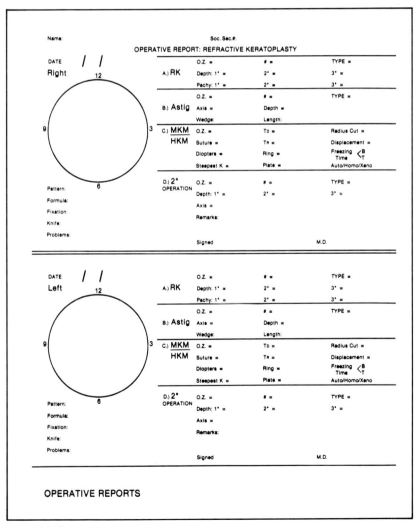

Figure 4-17D.

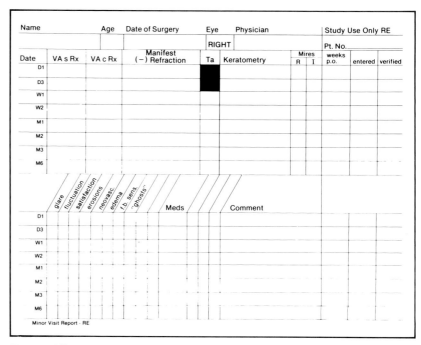

Figure 4-17E.

developed by Blackwell, Gravenstein and Kaufman,[42] is essentially a modification of a long light rod calibrated in degrees over which the eye must rotate to fixate on a small rheostat-controlled bulb. This fixation device allows precise location of the areas of photography in a consistent manner. It also provides a more sensitive method of detecting early regional cell loss from the refractive keratoplasty procedures. The use of the specular microscope is limited in the average clinical practice due to the expense of the instrumentation as well as the expense and time to the patient. Nevertheless, it must be remembered that the failure, long term, of previous incisional refractive keratoplasty was due to endothelial decompensation over a period of 20 years after initially uncomplicated surgery. Although the initial studies in endothelial counts in radial keratotomy are guardedly positive, a potential time bomb still exists. Only with thorough regional assessment of endothelial cell counts, preoperatively and postoperatively, accounting for incisional depth, location and complications, will the true effect of corneal incisions upon the endothelium be validly assessed.

Conclusion. Radial keratotomy today is as much an art as a science. The engineering analysis of the cornea and the predicted effects of radial incisions are theoretically useful but not at present clinically applicable. Statistically derived nomograms or equations, although imprecise, are the best means at present for predicting surgical effect. No method is universally accepted because of variation in surgical technique, but the surgeon must settle upon one to acquire consistent results. The key to using a nomogram or equation is to carefully note the technique of the investigator upon whose work this is derived. With continued research (Figure 4-17) and database management, the individual surgeon can modify his system based upon prior experience. Until one universal surgical technique is adopted, only diligent analysis by the individual surgeon can refine the confidence intervals of each surgical parameter.

References

1. Fyodorov SN, Agranovsky AA: Long-Term Results of Anterior Radial Keratotomy. *J Ocul Ther Surg:* 217-223, July-Aug, 1982.
2. Bores LD: Radial Keratotomy: A progress report of the American experience. *Ophthalmic Forum* 1:24-27, 1982.
3. Rowsey JJ, Balyeat HD: Preliminary Results and Complications of Radial Keratotomy. *Am J Ophthalmol* 93:437-455, 1982.
4. Hoffer KJ, Darin JJ, Pettit TH, et al: UCLA Clinical Trial of Radial Keratotomy: Preliminary report. *Ophthalmology* 88:729-736, 1981.
5. Arrowsmith P, Deitz M, Kremer F, et al: Analysis of Radial Keratotomy. Interim Report. Study Group, presented at Keratorefractive Society Meeting, November, 1982, San Francisco, CA.
6. Stark WJ, Martin NF, et al: Radial Keratotomy, A Risk Procedure of Unproven Long Term Success. *Surv Ophthalmol* 28:101-111, 1983.
7. Schachar RA, Black TD, Huang T: *Understanding Radial Keratotomy.* Denison, TX: LAL Publishing, 1981, pp 201-225.
8. Arrowsmith PN: A Mark Software, 1983.
9. Kremer F: Accutome, Inc., 1983.
10. Duane TD, Jaeger EA: Clinical Ophthalmology. Philadelphia: Harper and Row, Vol 1, Chapt 60, 1981.
11. Doss D, Hutson RL, Rowsey JJ: Method for Calculation of Corneal Profile and Power Distribution. *Arch Ophthalmol* 99:1261, 1981.
12. Rowsey JJ: Corneal Topography: Corneascope. *Arch Ophthalmol* 99:1093, 1981.
13. Corneascope; International Diagnostic Instrument's Corneascope; Broken Arrow, OK.
14. Kerascan Keratograph Autoanalyzer, KERA Corporation; Mountain View, CA.
15. Nordan LT: *Current Status of Refractive Surgery.* San Diego: CL Printing, 1983.
16. Bailey IL, Lovie JE: New Design Principles for Visual Acuity Charts. *Am J Optom Physiol Opt* 53:740, 1976.
17. Diabetic Retinopathy Study Research Group. Report #6: Design, methods and baseline results. *Invest Ophthalmol Vis Sci* 21:149, 1981.
18. Sloan LL: Needs for Precise Measures of Acuity Equipment to Meet These Needs: *Arch Ophthalmol* 98:286, 1980.
19. Schachar RA, Black TD: A Physicist's View of Radial Keratotomy; Keratorefraction. Denison, TX: LAL Publishing, 195-220, 1980.
20. Langhaar HL: *Foundations of Practical Shell Analysis.* Chicago: Univ. of Illinois, 1964.
21. Kobayashi AS, Woo LY: Analysis of the Corneo-scleral Shell by the Method of Direct Stiffness: *J Biomechanics* 4:323, 1971.
22. Mow CC: A Theoretical Model of the Cornea for Use in Studies of Tonometry. *Bull Math Biophysics* 301:437, 1968.
23. Schwartz MJ, Mackay RS: A Theoretical and Experimental Study of the Mechanical Behavior of the Cornea with Application to the Measurement of Intraocular Pressure. *Bull Math Biophysics* 28:585, 1966.
24. Love AEH: A Treatise on the Mathematical Theory of Elasticity. New York: Dover Publications, 1944, p 142.
25. Friedenwald JS: Contribution to the Theory and Practice of Tonometry. *Am J Ophthalmol* 20:985, 1937.
26. Hecht SD, Jamara RJ: Prospective Evaluation of Radial Keratotomy Using the Fyodorov Formula: Preliminary report. *Ann Ophthalmol* 14:319-330, 1982.
27. Hecht SD: Usefulness of Maklakov Tonometry to Predict Radial Keratotomy Outcome. Read before Keratorefractive Society, Chicago, 1983.
28. Mishima S, Hedbys BO: Measurement of Corneal Thickness with the Haag-Streit Pachymeter. *Arch Ophthalmol* 80:710-713, 1981.

29. Green DG: Corneal Thickness Measured by Interferometry. *J Optical Soc Am* 65:119, 1975.

30. Salz JJ, Azen SP, et al: Evaluation and Comparison of Sources of Variability in the Measurement of Corneal Thickness with Ultrasonic and Optical Pachymeters. *Ophth Surgery* 14:750-754, 1983.

31. Villasenor RA, Salz JJ: Changes in Corneal Thickness During Radial Keratotomy. *Ophthal Surg* 12:341-342, 1981.

32. Miller DA, Miller R: Glare Sensitivity in Simulated Radial Keratotomy. *Arch Ophthalmol* 99:1961-1962, 1981.

33. Miller D, Jernigan MS, Molnar S, et al: Laboratory Evaluation of a Clinical Glare Tester. *Arch Ophthalmol* 87:324-332, 1972.

34. LeClaire J, Nadler MP, Weiss J, et al: A New Glare Tester for Clinical Testing. *Arch Ophthalmol* 100: 1982.

35. Binder PS, Stainer GA, Zavala EY, et al: Acute Morphologic Features of Radial Keratotomy. *Arch Ophthalmol* 101:1113-1116, 1983.

36. Wright MR, Wright WK: A Psychological Study of Patient Undergoing Cosmetic Surgery. *Arch Otolaryngol* 101:145-151, 1975.

37. Waring GO, Moffit SD, Gelender H, et al: Rationale For and Design of the National Eye Institute Prospective Evaluation of Radial Keratotomy [PERK] Study. *Ophthalmol* 90:40-58, 1983.

38. Ware JE, Davies-Avery A: The Measurement and Meaning of Patient Satisfaction. *Health and Medical Care Services Review* 1:3-15, 1978.

39. Jester JV, Steel D, Salz J, et al: Radial Keratotomy in Non-human Primate Eyes. *Am J Ophthalmol* 92:153-171, 1981.

40. Hoffer KJ, Darrin JJ: The Effect of Radial Keratotomy on Axial Length and Endothelial Population in the Human. Read before the American Academy of Ophthalmology, Chicago, Nov. 7, 1980.

41. Hull DS, Farkas S, Green K: Radial Keratotomy: Effect on Corneal and Aqueous Humor Physiology in the Rabbit. *Arch Ophthalmol* 101:479-481, 1983.

42. Blackwell WL, Gravenstein N, Kaufman HE: Comparison of Central Corneal Endothelial Cell Numbers with Peripheral Areas. *Am J Ophthalmol* 84:473, 1977.

43. Bourque LB, Rubenstein MS, Cosand B, et al: Psychosocial Characteristics of Candidates for the Prospective Evaluation of Radial Keratotomy (PERK) Study. *Arch Ophthalmol* 102:1187-1192.

Chapter 5

Factors Affecting Predictability of Radial Keratotomy

Donald R. Sanders, MD, PhD
Michael R. Deitz, MD

FACTORS AFFECTING PREDICTABILITY OF RADIAL KERATOTOMY

Information concerning the patient-related and surgery-related factors which significantly affect the amount of correction obtained with radial keratotomy have come from original work by Fyodorov[1]; a number of experimental studies on animals and cadaver eyes (see Salz, Chapter 6); clinical observations by Thornton[2] and other surgeons in the United States; and statistical analysis of radial keratotomy data using such techniques as multiple regression analysis.[3]

The purpose of this chapter is to describe the factors believed to significantly affect refractive outcome of radial keratotomy and to present guidelines for estimating keratorefractive correction on an individual case basis. Because a great deal of work still needs to be done to refine and to further quantify the effect of various factors on refractive outcome, the information presented is approximate, but necessarily reflects some personal opinion based on reviewing large amounts of information.

Optical Zone Size

The zone size of the optical clear zone selected by the surgeon is the single most important factor determining refractive change in radial keratotomy. Deitz et al.[3] determined through regression analysis that 28% of the variability in refractive outcome at one year after radial keratotomy could be explained by differences in optical zone size. Within the range of 3.0 mm to 4.5 mm optical clear zone, reduction of the optical zone size by 0.5 mm resulted in slightly less than 1.0 diopters of additional myopia correction on the average. This approximately 2:1 ratio between myopia correction in diopters and optical zone size in mm has also been found by Thornton.[2] In the smaller optical zone size range (3.25 mm or less), decreases in optical zone size may possibly result in much larger changes in refractive outcome. Evidence for this is the reported case of marked overcorrection due to inadvertent surgical incursion into the central clear zone.[4] It is likely that with larger clear zones (above 4.5 mm), as the clear zone is increased even further, refractive effect may drop off rapidly.

Incision Depth

The exact mathematical relationship between incision depth and refractive outcome is unknown primarily due to the difficulties in accurately measuring incision depth. Nevertheless, there is little doubt that deeper corneal incisions result in more refractive effect. Jester et al in a series of studies on cadaver eyes[5] demonstrated that the most important factor in producing significant corneal flattening was depth of the incision. Deitz et al[3] found that incision depth was second only in importance to optical clear zone and could explain 16% of the variability in refractive outcome at one year. Using an average 90% incision depth at the optical zone, (measured by optical pachymetry postoperatively), Deitz achieved an average correction in myopia of 5.0 diopters at one year; results were stable by one month. This finding is in contradistinction to the work of Nirankiri et al[6] where average incision depth of close to 50% resulted in much less refractive change.

Kogan[7] has recently advocated shallow incision radial keratotomy as a means of providing a "safer" operation. Salz[8] has criticized this approach stating that prediction of refractive outcome becomes difficult and no reasonable surgical approach to the undercorrected patient remains available.

Determining just how to attain the desired incision depth may also be a problem since ultrasonic pachymetry instruments differ in design and calibration as do diamond knives and the gauge blocks used to assess blade extension. Because of these variations, the surgeon must "titrate" (i.e., individualize) his method of setting his diamond knife based on ultrasonic pachymetry to obtain his desired corneal incision depth.

Peripheral Re-deepening

It is difficult to see how deepening the most peripheral portion of an incision would increase refractive effect since the incision depth at the optical zone seems to be the most critical factor (see Chapter 6, Salz). Nevertheless, some surgeons have claimed to be able to increase effect by 0.5 diopters to 1.5 diopters by deepening the peripheral portions of the incisions.[2] Care must be taken with this approach because deepening the peripheral portion of the incision frequently results in corneal perforation.

Patient Age and Sex

It is a well known clinical phenomenon that older patients show more effect for the same amount of surgery than younger ones. In addition, our studies have revealed that young females do not receive as much refractive effect for the same amount of surgery as young males; this difference tends to diminish with age. A 20-year-old female achieves approximately 0.5 diopters less effect for the same surgical procedure as an equivalent 20-year-old male. This difference in effect between males and females is negligible by age 40. It is interesting to speculate that possibly these differences could be related to hormonal influences on collagen and that with the aging process the hormonal differences beween men and women decrease.

We have found in our regression analysis studies that patients achieve between 0.25 diopters to 0.50 diopters more effect per decade of age, this age-related effect being more prominent in females. Thus, a 40-year-old female patient could expect 1.0 diopters more myopia correction than a similar 20-year-old patient given the same amount of surgery whereas a male patient could expect approximately 0.5 diopters more effect with increasing age. This age-related increase may be due to an increase in scleral rigidity.

Number of Incisions

The refractive effect of varying the number of incisions in animal and cadaver eyes has been summarized in detail by Salz in Chapter 6. We have found that a 16-incision radial keratotomy increases the effect of an eight-incision case by approximately 0.5 diopters to 1.5 diopters, assuming a 3 mm optical zone size. We believe that the use of 16-incision radial keratotomy should be reserved for cases with 3 mm optical zones that require somewhat more correction than can be expected with eight incisions. Others have suggested the effect of an additional eight incisions at the time of surgery can be as much as 1.75 diopters to 2.0 diopters. Rowsey has shown less effect with 16 incisions than with eight incisions.[9] As Salz has pointed out, the amount of additional effect in a 16-incision case may depend on the depth of the original eight incisions.

Recently a number of surgeons have advocated performing a two-staged radial keratotomy beginning with four incisions in the first operation. If the patient is undercorrected, an additional four incisions are performed at a later date. One value of this approach is to minimize overcorrections since four incisions alone may completely correct the patient and no further surgery need be performed. It has been the experience of one of the Editors that the maximum obtainable long-term correction from four incisions with a 3 mm optical zone is 3.0 diopters.

Intraocular Pressure

It is generally believed that a higher postoperative intraocular pressure results in more refractive effect with radial keratotomy. Some surgeons even advocate the use of steroids in undercorrected individuals to induce an increase in intraocular pressure and thus a greater effect (Figure 5-1). We have found that preoperative intraocular pressure measurements may have some slight predictive value. With all other factors being equal, a patient with a preoperative intraocular pressure of 20 mm Hg could expect to obtain as much as 0.25 to 0.5 diopters more effect from the same amount of surgery as a patient with a preoperative tension of 10 mm Hg. Thornton believes that the effect of surgery is lessened with preoperative pressures below 11 mm Hg and enhanced with pressures above 19 mm Hg.[2]

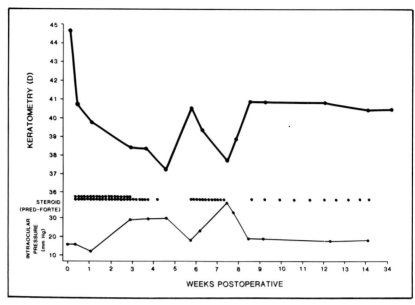

Figure 5-1. Relationship between surgically-induced corneal flattening as measured by keratometry and intraocular pressure following radial keratometry. Topical steroids induced an intraocular pressure rise which correlated with an increased flattening of the cornea. (Data courtesy of Dr. Michael Deitz.)

Preoperative Average Keratometry

One can expect a slightly greater effect from the same amount of surgery in a patient with a steep cornea than in a patient with a flat cornea. The difference in refractive effect amounts to only about 1 diopter within the physiologic range of preoperative keratometry measurements from 42 to 46 diopters.

Corneal Diameter

We have found a slightly greater effect of surgery in patients with larger corneal diameters. This amounts to only a 0.25 diopters difference in effect within the normal range of corneal diameters.

Determination of Operative Parameters

Given a patient's preoperative characteristics (age, sex, refractive error, keratometry, intraocular pressure, and corneal diameter) the radial keratotomy surgeon must formulate a surgical plan to attempt to correct a patient's refractive problem. In general, the surgeon must decide the size and shape of the central optical clear zone, and the number, depth, length, and placement of incisions to be performed.

A number of tables, nomograms, and equations have been developed which claim to provide guidelines for predictable surgery. In general, given the amount of myopia to be corrected, these guides tell the surgeon how large an optical zone to use, and how many and how deep the incisions should be made. The various methods differ in the number of other patient-related factors taken into account (i.e., patient age, sex, pre-operative intraocular pressure, keratometry, and corneal diameter) and whether peripheral re-deepening incisions are recommended. None of these surgical guides have been tested for accuracy in a large series of cases performed by multiple surgeons. Therefore, the general applicability of any of them is uncertain.

The nomogram and explanatory material reproduced in Appendix 5-1 outline the surgical approach of Dr. Michael Deitz. The nomogram and modifying factors described are a simplification and clinical modification of the equation derived by statistical analysis of a large series of radial keratotomy cases. The equation is available for use with a Texas Instruments CC-40 calculator/computer and printer and will be incorporated in a number of new ultrasonic pachymetry devices being produced. Formulas developed by Fyodorov and Bores will be similarly available. Since, as has been mentioned, none of the methods for predicting the amount of surgery to be performed has been extensively tested for universal applicability, they all should be viewed as general guidelines that must be modified based on the surgeon's own results. Indeed, the Deitz equation and that of Fyodorov and Bores are being developed to allow surgeons to tailor the formulas based on their own results, similar to the individual tailoring of "A" constants for the SRK formula used in intraocular lens implant power calculation.

The Thornton Guide for Radial Keratotomy Incisions and Optical Zone Size reproduced in Appendix 5-2 is based on retrospective clinical reviews of many hundreds of cases. This guide is also being programmed for simplified use with the CC-40 computer.

References

1. Fyodorov SN: Radial Keratotomy, *In* Schachar RA, Levy NS, Schachar L (eds). *Refractive Modulation of the Cornea: Proceedings of the Annual Keratorefractive Society Meeting on Radial Keratotomy and Keratorefraction.* Denison, TX: LAL Publishing, 1981, pp 89-120.
2. Thornton SP: *Thornton Guide for Radial Keratotomy Incisions and Optical Zone Size.* Nashville, TN: Spencer Thornton, 1981.
3. Deitz MR, Sanders DR, Marks RG: Radial Keratotomy: An overview of the Kansas City study. *Ophthalmology* 1984; 91:467-478.
4. Arrowsmith PN, Sanders DR, Marks RG: Visual, refractive and keratometric results of radial keratotomy. *Arch Ophthalmol* 1983; 101:873-881.
5. Jester J, Venet T, Lee J, et al: A Statistical Analysis of Radial Keratotomy in Human Cadaver Eyes. *Am J Ophthalmol* 1981; 92:172-177.
6. Nirankiri VS, Katzen LE, Richards RD, et al: Prospective Clinical Study of Radial Keratotomy. *Ophthalmology* 1982; 89:677-683.
7. Kogan L: Advantages of shallow radial keratotomy incisions sited. *IOL & Ocular Surgery News* April 1, 1984; 2(7):1, 23.
8. Salz J: Thirty-two many. Editorial. *IOL & Ocular Surgery News* June 1, 1984; 2(11):4-5.
9. Rowsey JJ, Balyeat HD, Rabinovitch B, et al: Predicting the results of radial keratotomy. *Ophthalmology* 1983; 90:642-654.

Appendix 5-1

Deitz Nomogram for Determination of RK Operative Parameters

Basic philosophy. The basic philosophy underlying the Deitz nomogram is to approach the lowest myopia levels with eight single or primary incisions of approximately 86% to 90% depth. With greater degrees of myopia, the optical zone size is decreased to a minimum of 3.0 mm. The depth of the incision is the next parameter to be changed as higher myopia levels (5 diopters to 6 diopters) are attacked. A greater incision depth (91% to 93%) is achieved by recutting the radial incisions from optical zone to periphery using the same micrometer knife setting as with the primary incisions. If further correction is necessary, then the number of incisions is increased from 8 to 16.

Achieving the attempted incision depth. Using the Micra double-cutting diamond knife with flat footplate and the Kremer Corneometer I with velocity set at 1,640 m/s, the blade is set at the thinnest paracentral ultrasonic corneal thickness plus 0.03 mm. If Dr. Deitz makes a single pass through the incision at this setting, he achieves an 86% to 90% observed incision depth postoperatively. If he recuts the radial incisions without changing the blade settings, he achieves a 91% to 93% postoperative incision depth. Obviously, the pachymeter at this setting is reading the cornea as much thinner than it actually is, the blade setting is less than measured or the knife blade is going shallower than it is actually set.

The individual surgeon must "titrate" his pachymetry, knife setting, and surgical technique to obtain the desired postoperative incision depth.

Other modifying factors. Keratometry and Intraocular Pressure Preoperative keratometry measurements (K) less than 42 diopters or greater than 46 diopters, and intraocular pressures less than 12 mm Hg or greater than 23 mm Hg dictate adjustments in optical zone size. Flat corneas or low IOPs require more surgical correction so the optical zone size is decreased by 0.25 mm from that suggested by the nomogram for each of these conditions. Steep corneas or high IOPs require less surgical correction and the optical zone size is increased by 0.25 mm for each of these conditions. Adjustments for IOP and keratometry should be considered additive so that a case with a high K and high IOP would have 0.5 mm added to the optical zone. A case with flat K and high IOP would require no change from the nomograms with regard to optical zone size because the adjustments would cancel each other out. If any combination of flat K or low IOP dictates an optical zone size of less than 3.0 mm, then the incisions are recut to 91% to 93% depth. If this was already required, then the number of incisions are increased to 16. If this, in turn, was already required, then the patient may be a poor candidate for total correction of myopia.

DEITZ NOMOGRAM FOR RK PARAMETERS

Correction Required (Diopters)	Patient Age	Male			Female		
		Number of Primary Incisions	Clear Zone	Attempted Incision Depth (%)†	Number of Primary Incisions	Clear Zone	Attempted Incision Depth (%)†
1.00	20	8	5.30	86-90	8	4.8	86-90
	40	8	5.70	86-90	8	5.5	86-90
1.50	20	8	5.10	86-90	8	4.5	86-90
	40	8	5.40	86-90	8	5.3	86-90
2.00	20	8	4.80	86-90	8	4.3	86-90
	40	8	5.20	86-90	8	5.0	86-90
2.50	20	8	4.50	86-90	8	4.0	86-90
	40	8	5.00	86-90	8	4.8	86-90
3.00	20	8	4.80	86-90	8	3.7	86-90
	40	8	4.60	86-90	8	4.5	86-90
3.50	20	8	4.00	86-90	8	3.5	86-90
	40	8	4.40	86-90	8	4.8	86-90
4.00	20	8	3.70	86-90	8	3.2	86-90
	40	8	4.40	86-90	8	4.0	86-90
4.50	20	8	3.50	86-90	8	3.0	86-90
	40	8	3.80	86-90	8	3.7	86-90
5.00	20	8	3.20	86-90	8	3.0	91-93†
	40	8	3.60	86-90	8	3.4	86-90
5.50	20	8	3.00	86-90	16	3.0	91-93†
	40	8	3.30	86-90	8	3.2	86-90
6.00	20	8	3.00	91-93†	*	*	*
	40	8	3.00	86-90	8	3.2	91-93†
7.00	20	*	*	*	*	*	*
	40	16	3.00	91-93†	*	*	*
8.00	20	*	*	*	*	*	*
	40	*	*	*	*	*	*
9.00	20	*	*	*	*	*	*
	40	*	*	*	*	*	*

*These patients have parameters of myopia, age, and sex that theoretically would require the maximum number of incisions (16) at maximum depth (91% to 93%) and optical zone sizes of less than 3.0 mm to achieve emmetropia. Because decreasing optical zone size below 3.0 mm would increase the possibility of symptomatic glare, these patients must be considered poorer candidates for total or optimal correction. With more advanced surgical techniques, some experienced surgeons may be able to achieve greater effect; however, this is not recommended for beginning radial keratotomy surgeons. It should be borne in mind that at any time when deeper incision depths are achieved, significantly greater effect is obtained.

†See discussion on Deitz nomogram, subsection "Achieving Attempted Incision Depth."

Appendix 5-2

Thornton Guide for Radial Keratotomy Incisions and Optical Zone Size

(A Simplified Method for Calculating the Procedure To Correct A Given Refractive Error With Eight or 16 Incisions)

After using the Fyodorov Nomograms for more than a year on a large number of cases, this guide was developed and subsequently revised over a period of several years based on periodic "best fit" review of many hundreds of cases.

This guide is designed to provide a simple method of producing a predictable radial keratotomy correction without a computer or complicated calculations. Necessary to understanding the steps to calculating a predictable correction of radial keratotomy is a basic understanding of terms. Each eye is different with many variables such as refractive error, corneal curvature, corneal diameter, thickness of cornea, and so forth. The only factors that can be varied in the surgical procedure are the optical zone, depth of incision, number, and pattern of incisions.

Instead of plotting a number of nomograms which introduce further variables, I have chosen to follow one specific set of guidelines which have produced consistently good results for me. The object of this guide is to provide maximum correction with the largest possible optical zone. For the experienced radial keratotomy surgeon, the optical zone can be enlarged by 0.25 mm in errors of up to −5.0 diopters (that is from 3.0 to 3.25 or 3.75 to 4.0, and so forth) by redeepening all incisions to 95% of pachymetric thickness from a point 2 mm from the optical zone margin. I recommend however that until one is quite experienced that he use this guide precisely.

Incisions should be carried to the limbus; that is, through the limbal arcade but not through the limbal junction. In practical terms this means to carry the incision to within 0.5 mm from the anatomic limbus.

The term "differential redeepening" means redeepening to Descemet's membrane throughout the length of the incision.

For this guide to produce the corrections for myopia and astigmatism noted on the chart with maximal effect and minimal regression, you must use a primary incision depth of 98% of the corneal thickness as measured at the optical zone margin (if the optical zone margin is at 3 mm it should be 98% of the depth at 3 mm. If the optical zone margin is at 4 mm the blade should be set at 98% of the depth at that point, not at the 3 mm optical zone margin.)

Modifiers. Modifiers are those factors which necessitate a modification of the myopic power to be corrected. **Believe the Modifiers.** Calculate your modifiers before determining the optical zone from the Guide.

Age. The Thornton "2% Rule" for Modification of RK

Effect by Age. "For every year *below* age 30 *add 2%* to the myopic error." "For every year *above* age 30 *subtract 2%* from the myopic error to age 40, then 1% per year to age 50 and ½% per year thereafter."

The Female Factor. If your patient is female reduce the age by three years. Women's eyes act as if they are three years younger than men's. Before calculation of myopic error subtract three years from the age if female.

The Intraocular Pressure Rule. "For every mm below 11 add 3% to the myopic refractive error. For every mm above 19, subtract 3% from the myopic refractive error."

Low Astigmatism (Up To 2.5 Diopters). In myopic astigmatism use the following steps:
1. Add the spherical equivalent of astigmatism up to 0.75 diopters to the myopic error.
2. With astigmatism over 0.75 diopters add the spherical equivalent up to 0.75 diopters to the myopia and correct the remainder with T or L procedures.
3. If the remainder is under 1.5 diopters, *rotate* the incisions so that the axis of correction of astigmatism is between the incisions. If the astigmatism is over 1.5 diopters, make corrective T cuts across the radial incisions.

Using the Modifiers. All modifiers result in a percentage change of the refractive error. The modifiers must be totaled and the percentage change added or subtracted to the patient's myopia before referring to the Guide. Once you have added or subtracted the percentage error as determined by your modifiers use this theoretic myopic error as if it were the actual myopic error of your patient. Locate this amount of myopia along the top of the Guide, then look down the side of the guide to the keratometry reading and at the junction of those two columns you will find the optical zone necessary.

To get the effect predicted and desired, you must use essentially the same technique as suggested by the author. I use diamond blade incisions carried from the optical zone to the limbus beginning with a 98% depth and redeepen my incisions to 95% depth as measured by pachymetry in the periphery where indicated. Using a technique different from my method will of course yield different results.

Thornton Guide for Optical Zone Size

Myopia	1.50 – 2.00	2.12 – 2.50	2.62 – 3.00	3.12 – 3.62	3.74 – 4.25	4.37 – 5.00	5.12 – 6.00	6.12 – 8.00	>8.00
Keratometry									
40.00-42.00	4.00	3.75	3.50	3.25	3.00	3.00 re-deepen peripheral 1/3	3.00 re-deepen peripheral 1/2	3.00 16 cuts re-deepen 1/2	3.00 16 cuts differential re-deepen
42.12-44.00	4.25	4.00	3.75	3.50	3.25	3.00	3.00 re-deepen peripheral 1/3	3.00 16 cuts	3.00 16 cuts differential re-deepen ½
44.12-46.25	4.50	4.25	4.00	3.75	3.50	3.25	3.00	3.00 re-deepen peripheral ½	3.00 16 cuts re-deepen peripheral ½ of 8 cuts
46.37-48.00	4.75	4.50	4.25	4.00	3.75	3.50	3.25	3.00	3.00 16 cuts re-deepen peripheral ½ of 8 cuts

NOTE: Redeepening for higher powers should be carried to 95% of corneal thickness as measured by pachymetry in the mid-periphery and periphery (i.e. essentially to Descemet's).

"Peripheral 1/3" = Begin cuts 2.5 mm from the 3 mm optical zone margin and carry to the limbus that is, use an 8 mm optical zone for the deepening cuts.
"Peripheral 1/2" = Begin cuts 1.5 mm from the 3 mm optical zone margin and carry to the limbus that is, use a 6 mm optical zone for the deepening cuts.

Chapter 6

Pathophysiology of Radial Keratotomy Incisions

James J. Salz, MD

PATHOPHYSIOLOGY OF RADIAL KERATOTOMY INCISIONS

The present chapter attempts to summarize the available clinical and experimental data about the pathophysiology of radial keratotomy incisions. The discussion focuses on the proper number of radial keratotomy (RK) incisions, their length and depth, the manner in which they heal, and their effect on the corneal endothelium.

Number of Radial Keratotomy Incisions

The first report in the American literature about radial keratotomy incisions was by Sato[1] of Japan in 1953. He utilized up to 40 anterior incisions combined with about 32 posterior incisions. In 1979 Fyodorov[2] concluded that the proper number of incisions was 16, all anterior.

Eight Versus 16 Incisions. The refractive surgery group at U.S.C. approached the question of the ideal number of incisions by studying the effect of varying numbers of incisions in human cadaver eyes and in owl and stump tail monkeys.[3-6] We found that about 60% of the effect of a 16 incision radial keratotomy in a cadaver eye takes place with the first four incisions. Adding four more incisions generally adds another 30% and placing the final eight incisions only adds another 10%. Thus if making 16 incisions flattens a cadaver cornea 10 diopters, the first four incisions will produce 6 diopters, the next four incisions will produce an additional 3 diopters, and the final eight incisions usually add only another 1 diopters.

Since the cadaver eye is a static system there is of course no regression of effect. We tested our conclusion about the potential advantages of eight-incision RK on two groups of monkeys. There was no significant difference in the final amount of corneal flattening induced by eight versus 16 incisions.

Dr. Ronald Smith at USC stimulated a group of graduate students at the California Institute of Technology to devise a mechanical model of the cornea. Under the direction of Dr. Wolfgang Knaus, they studied the effects of 4, 8, 16, and 32 incisions on a pressurized corneal model made of a plastic polymer, solithane.[7] Their findings were in general agreement with our results from the cadaver and monkey studies.

Dr. Ronald Schachar, who is a physicist in addition to being an ophthalmologist, developed a complicated theoretical model of the cornea.[8] Independent of our cadaver eye studies, he accurately predicted that eight-incision radial keratotomy would produce almost 90% of the effect of 16 incisions.

TABLE 6-1
Summary of Corneal Flattening in Diopters Per # of Incisions Cadaver
Eyes—4.0 mm. Optical Clear Zone

# of Incisions	Corneal Flattening in Diopers
3	5.08
4	6.80
6	8.20
8	9.50
12	9.13
16	9.00

Note: The 16 incision data were based on metal blade incisions set at 90% of optical pachymetry. All the others were performed with micrometer diamond knives set at 100% of ultrasonic pachymetry. There were 6 eyes in each group.

IMPORTANT! THIS TABLE IS NOT A NOMOGRAM DESIGNED FOR CLINICAL USE

Clinical reports by Rowsey,[9] Hoffer,[10] and Nirankari,[11] have validated the experimental data cited above by proving the effectiveness of eight-incision radial keratotomy in controlled studies. Nirankari's report also addressed the issue of adding eight additional incisions to three patients who were undercorrected after their first eight incisions. Two of these patients actually became slightly more myopic following their second surgery. I have recently reviewed the effect of adding eight additional incisions in 14 patients in my own series. In 11 patients where the original incisions were graded at greater than 80% depth, adding eight additional incisions resulted in only about 1 diopter of additional effect. In three patients where the incisions were less than 80% depth, the second surgery added an average of about 2 diopter of additional refractive effect. This suggests that if the original eight incisions are of adequate depth, adding eight more is unlikely to be beneficial and may in fact be harmful.

Four Incisions. Since our research indicated that most of the effect of a radial keratotomy occurs after the first four incisions, we decided to apply this principle to selected patients. The results have been most encouraging. A preliminary report on my experience with four-incision RK was presented at the Keratorefractive Society meeting in Chicago in November, 1983. Four-incision RK with a 3.0 mm. optical zone in five eyes resulted in 3.5 diopter of refractive change. In eight other eyes, four-incision RK with a 3.5 mm. optical zone produced 2.56 diopter of refractive change. All patients have been followed for over six months and the longest followup is over two years. Dr. James Rowsey in Oklahoma is following a group of patients who underwent four-incision RK with a 3.0 mm. optical zone and are averaging almost 5 diopter of refractive correction (personal communication) in short term followup.

The apparent discrepancy between my results and Rowsey's in patients with a 3.0 mm. optical zone is probably explained by differences in patient selection and use of postoperative topical cortisone. I performed four-incision RK on patients who were from 2.0 to 3.5 diopter myopic and I did not routinely use cortisone. Rowsey is attempting to study the maximum correction that can be achieved by four incisions so he is selecting more myopic patients and placing all of them on postoperative cortisone drops.

Six and 12 Incisions. Some surgeons have begun to study the effects of six- and 12-incision RK.[12] I reviewed the results of three-, six-, and 12-incision RK in a series of five cadaver eyes (unpublished data) with the surgery being performed in a manner similar to our other studies.[3,4] The induced keratometric corneal flattening was as follows: three incisions—5.08 diopters six incisions—8.20 diopter, 12 incisions—9.13 diopter. Once again it is apparent that most of the effect occurs after the first three incisions and very little is gained by the last six. Since we averaged 6.8 diopter after four incisions and 9.5 diopter after eight incisions[4] it would seem that there is little advantage to trying to titrate the effect of RK by adopting a three-, six-, 12-pattern instead of four or eight. The proper spacing of these incisions is more difficult and it would introduce another variable into the analysis of RK results which is already challenging enough.

Table 6-1 summarizes the induced corneal flattening in cadaver eyes per number of incisions utilizing a 4.0 mm clear zone.

Incision Length

To Limbus Versus Through Limbus. Sato's original article on RK described a large number of relatively short incisions, utilizing an optical zone of about 6.0 mm.[1] Fyodorov reported much better results with far fewer strictly anterior incisions by making longer incisions closer to the optical center of the cornea.[2] He originally advised extending these incisions past the limbus in order to cut the "circular ligament of the cornea" and he introduced the concept of changing the size of the optical clear zone as a method of titrating the effect of RK.

Numerous clinical reports[9,10,13] have validated the concept of adjusting the size of the clear zone for the degree of myopia. Our latest study on cadaver eyes demonstrates the decreasing effect of RK as the optical zone increases from 3 mm to 6 mm (Submitted for publication—CLAO Journal). For example, eight-incision RK with a 6.0 mm optical zone produced only 2.29 diopter of corneal flattening, whereas a 3.0 mm zone produces almost 9.0 diopter of effect.

As to the "circular ligament," the work at U.S.C. on cadaver and monkey eyes demonstrated that incisions through the limbus at times entered the trabecular meshwork and were slightly less effective in altering corneal curvature than incisions stopping in clear cornea.[3,5,6] Schachar[8] and Knauss[9] reached the same conclusion from a physicist's viewpoint.

Short Incisions. Based on his theoretical model of the cornea,

Schachar suggests that performing very short mid-peripheral incisions can be just as effective as those that stop at the limbus.[14] Our work in cadaver eyes has shown that although this was true in some eyes, most eyes attained significantly more effect when the incisions were extended to the limbus.[4,5] We have had no actual clinical experience with these short incisions.

Incision Depth

Metal Blades and Optical Pachymetry. Most radial keratotomy surgeons feel that deep incisions are probably the most critical aspect of the operation. Jester performed a detailed statistical analysis on our cadaver eye work and found that the most important factor in producing significant corneal flattening was the depth of the incision.[16] Our original studies showed considerable variation in incision depth[4,5] when surgery was performed with metal blade settings based on optical pachymetry (Figure 6.1).

Micrometer Diamond Knives and Ultrasonic Pachymetry. The introduction of micrometer diamond knives and ultrasonic pachymetry seems to offer the intrumentation necessary to achieve more consistent incision depth. A histologic analysis of RK incisions in cadaver eyes utilizing the surgical technique and instrumentation recommended in the PERK study[17] demonstrated histologically confirmed incision depths of 80% to 90% along the entire length of the majority of the incisions with both metal and diamond blades (Figure 6.2). Our clinical experience has

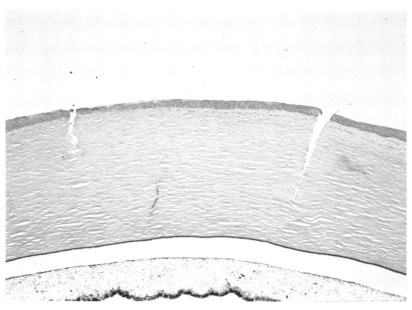

Figure 6-1.

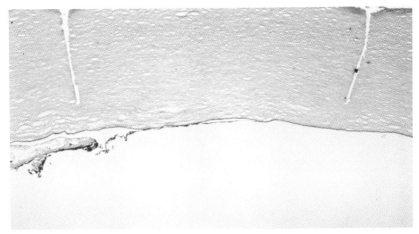

Fig. 6-2. More consistent incision depth following RK in a cadaver eye. Micrometer diamond knife setting based on ultrasonic pachymetry.

been that this technique produces consistently deep incisions from the optical zone to the peripheral cornea with an extremely low incidence of perforations.

Stepped Incisions and Re-deepening. Some surgeons have emphasized the importance of "stepped" incisions or "peripheral re-deepening"[12,18,19] when larger amounts of correction are desired. This is a difficult concept to prove conclusively without knowing how much effect a given eye might have attained without the re-deepening. Comparing the results of eyes operated on previously without the re-deepening, either in the same patients or other patients, introduces the additional variable of improved surgical technique with the surgeon's increased experience. Thus an apparent improvement in results following re-deepening may have occurred even with a single incision technique due to the surgeon's increased experience.

From a theoretical standpoint, the concept of re-deepening the peripheral portion of the incision is troublesome. Most experts would agree that the majority of the effect of RK is caused by the portion of the incision closest to the optical zone. This point is validated by the clinical reports which demonstrate the increasing effect of the operation as the incisions approach the optical center of the cornea. Why should re-deepening the peripheral portion of the incision, for example from the 6.0 mm zone to the periphery, be expected to improve the result? A recent study in our laboratory (unpublished data) on 24 cadaver eyes failed to demonstrate a significant increase in the effect of RK following peripheral re-deepening but did dramatically increase the perforation rate (Figure 6-3).

Templates and Fixation Rings. Since deep incisions are deemed critical for correcting the higher amounts of myopia, alternate methods of performing the incisions have been suggested. These approaches include the use of templates and suction rings.

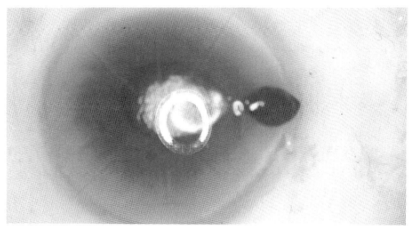

Fig. 6-3. Perforation with iris prolapse following peripheral re-deepening in a cadaver eye.

Both Kramer[20] and McIntyre[21] have suggested the template approach to RK. Kramer reported a method of making reproducible 0.5 mm incisions in pig corneas but this report lacked histologic validation. Since the pig cornea is greater than 1.0 mm thick, these incisions were only about half thickness and it remains to be seen whether consistent 90% incisions could be accomplished.

Gellender has recently published a report describing the advantages of a pneumatic fixation ring to help fixate the eye and stabilize the intraocular pressure while performing RK.[22] Although it is his impression that the ring is helpful, there is as yet no published independent clinical or experimental data to substantiate its value.

How Deep Can We Go? How deep can the radial keratotomy blade be safely set? Rowsey has recently shown that two of the most popular diamond knives, KOI and Micra, are already cutting about 20% deeper than the blade settings would indicate.[23] Despite this finding, setting these same knives at 100% of the thinnest paracentral ultrasonic pachymetry (velocity 1640) rarely results in perforation, whereas setting the blade at 110% almost always does (personal experience with six patients and five perforations). I found in a series of 10 cadaver eyes that perforations usually did not occur until the blade was advanced at least .06 mm greater than 100% of the underlying ultrasonic pachymeter reading. I have empirically added .04 to 100% of the thinnest reading in several cases without perforating.

How They Heal

Radial keratotomy incisions basically heal like other corneal incisions through the process of avascular wound healing.[5,6] During the first 48 hours, epithelium slides into the incision forming an epithelial plug. Over

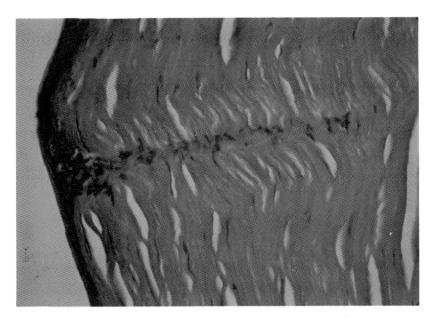

Figure 6-4. Monkey eye RK incision at three weeks. Fibroblasts have replaced epithelial plug along incision site.

Figure 6-5. Monkey eye RK incision at three months. Incision site identified only by break in Bowman's membrane and slight increase in keratocytes along incision line.

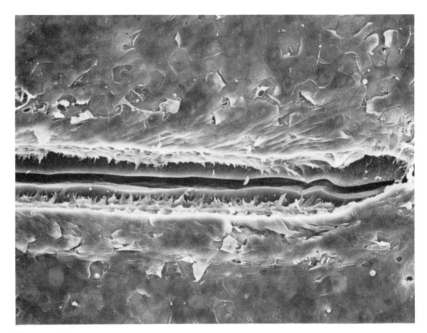

Figure 6-6A.

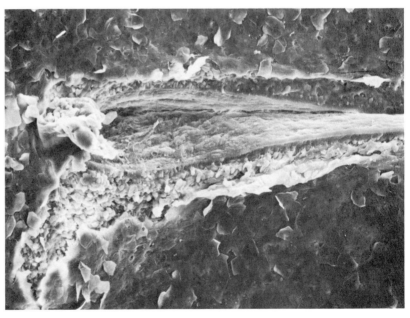

Figure 6-6B.

Fig. 6-6. Scanning electron micrographs of incisions made with metal razor blade fragments: A. Site of razor-blade entrance (×420). B. Site of razor-blade exit (×240). Photos courtesy of Perry S. Binder, M.D.

the next two weeks this plug is gradually replaced by fibroblasts (Figure 6-4). By the end of three months the fibroblasts have disappeared and the well healed incision site is barely identified by the disruption of Bowman's membrane and the presence of slightly more keratocytes in the area (Figure 6-5). Our study and a report by Binder[24] have demonstrated that the exit site where the RK blade is removed produces more trauma to Bowman's membrane than the entry site (Figure 6-6), a point in favor of initiating the incision at the optical zone rather than terminating the incision at the optical zone as Fyodorov advises. By completing the incision near the limbus, the area where the scarring is likely to be greater is further away from the optical axis. This should help minimize the glare from the incisions.

The Effects of Radial Keratotomy Incisions on the Endothelium

Acute Changes. Because of the high incidence of bullous keratopathy in Sato's patients,[25] one of the major concerns about RK is the possible effect on the endothelium. During the first 48 hours following RK in monkeys, inflammatory cells are seen along the endothelium and some vacuolation is apparent between cells at about two weeks. These changes gradually resolved, and except for individual cell loss, the endothelium remained essentially unchanged for the one year duration of the study.[6] A recent report by Hull demonstrated no significant alterations in corneal endothelial permeability following RK in rabbits as measured by fluorophotometry.[26]

Endothelial Cell Loss—Experimental. Eight-incision RK with metal blades in owl monkeys produced a mean 14% endothelial cell loss at six months.[6] We repeated the RK procedure utilizing a diamond knife in two other groups of monkeys, one group receiving post-operative cortisone and the other group receiving a placebo. We found no significant endothelial cell loss in either group (unpublished data). Yamaguchi reported no significant difference in endothelial cell loss (8% to 9%) in two groups of Green monkeys, one group treated with cortisone and the other with saline.[27] The two groups also ended up with about the same amount of corneal flattening. The cortisone treated owl monkeys in our study ended up with slightly more keratometric effect than the nontreated group. Rowsey has accumulated data which indicates that post-operative cortisone produces about 1 diopter of additional refractive effect and up to 2 diopter if the patient is a cortisone responder (personal communication).

Endothelial Cell Loss—Clinical. Clinical reports about the effect of RK on the endothelium seem to parallel the primate studies. Hoffer reported 10% endothelial cell loss following 16 incision RK at three months and 3% endothelial cell loss at six months following eight-incision RK.[10] Rowsey reported 7.6% cell loss following eight-incision RK at one year.[28]

Neither of these studies indicates that cell loss will be progressive following a single surgical procedure (based on a comparison of cell counts at three months which were repeated at one to two years in a small number of patients).

Repeat Surgery and the Endothelium. The question of endothelial cell damage following repeat radial keratotomy is another matter entirely. Six months after their original eight-incision RK, we placed eight additional incisions in our owl monkeys. There was no significant additional corneal flattening but they did lose an additional 10% of their endothelial cells. We repeated eight-incision RK every month for four months in one monkey and ended up with almost 30% cell loss. I have reported a similar cell loss in a patient following repeat radial keratotomy.[29] The wisdom of "touch up" operations and repeat radial keratotomy must be seriously questioned in light of the above observations. The cell loss appears to be caused by the surgical trauma and each insult to the cornea results in more cell loss.

Summary

Laboratory evaluation of the pathophysiology of radial keratotomy helps to answer many pertinent questions about the operation. The operation works well with eight and at times only four incisions that need not traverse the limbus. The concept of titrating the effect of the operation by varying the length of the incisions appears to be valid. Histologic confirmation that consistently deep incisions are possible with present instrumentation is now available. Although post-operative cortisone may enhance the effect of the operation, it does not appear to reduce endothelial cell loss. The radial incisions heal quite well and when the operation is properly performed there is very little damage to the endothelium in the short term. Repeat radial keratotomy and "touch up" operations should be approached with caution because of the potential for excessive cell loss and suggestive evidence that the additional incisions rarely produce a significant improvement in the refractive result.

References
1. Sato T, Akiyama K, Shibata H: A New Surgical Approach to Myopia. *Am J Ophthalmol* 36:823, 1953.
2. Fyodorov S, Durnev V: Operation of Dosaged Dissection of Corneal Circular Ligament in Cases of Myopia of Mild Degree. *Ann Ophthalmol* 11:1855, 1979.
3. Salz J, Lee J, Steel D, Villaseñor R, Nesburn A, Smith R: Radial Keratotomy in Fresh Human Cadaver Eyes. *Ophthalmol* 88:742, 1981.
4. Salz J, Lee T, Jester J, Villaseñor R, Steel D, Bernstein J, Smith R: Analysis of Incision Depth Following Experimental Radial Keratotomy. *Ophthalmol* 90:655, 1983.
5. Steel D, Jester J, Salz J, Villaseñor R, Lee T, Schanzlin D, Smith R: Modification of Corneal Curvature Following Radial Keratotomy in Primates. *Ophthalmol* 88:747, 1981.
6. Jester J, Steel D, Salz J, Miyoshiro J, Rife L, Schanzlin D, Smith R: Radial Keratotomy in Nonhuman Primates. *Am J Ophthalmol* 92:153, 1981.

7. Knauss W, Rapacz P, Sene K: Curvature Changes Induced by Radial Keratotomy in Solithane Model of Eye. *Invs Ophthal Vis Sci* (ARVO Abstract) 20(Suppl):69, 1982.

8. Schachar R, Black T, Huang T: A Physicist's View of Radial Keratotomy with Practical Surgical Implications. *In* RA Schachar, NS Levy and L Schachar, (eds), *Keratorefraction*. Denison, TX: LAL Publishing 1980. pp 195-220.

9. Rowsey J, Balyeat H, Rabinovitch B, Burris T, Hays J: Predicting the Results of Radial Keratotomy. *Ophthalmol* 90:642, 1983.

10. Hoffer K, Darin J, Pettit T, Hofbauer J, Elander R, Levenson J: Three Years Experience With Radial Keratotomy. *Ophthalmol* 90:627, 1983.

11. Nirankari V, Katzen L, Karesh J, Richards R, Lakhanpal V: Ongoing Prospective Clinical Study of Radial Keratotomy. *Ophthalmol* 90:637, 1983.

12. Bores L: Historical Review and Clinical Results of Radial Keratotomy. *Int Ophthalmol Clin* 23:93, 1983.

13. Bores L, Myers W, Cowden J: Radial Keratotomy: An analysis of the American experience. *Ann Ophthalmol* 13(8):941, 1981.

14. Schachar R, Black T, Huang T: Surgical Implications of the Theory of Radial Keratotomy. *In* RA Schachar, NS Levy, L Schachar (eds), *Radial Keratotomy*. Denison, TX: LAL Publishing, 1980. pp 269-286.

15. Salz J: Clinical Results of Radial Keratotomy in Fresh Human Cadaver Eyes. *In* RA Schachar, NS Levy, L Schachar (Eds), *Keratorefraction*. Denison, TX: LAL Publishing, 1980. pp 133-142.

16. Jester J, Venet T, Lee J, Schanzlin D, Smith R: A Statistical Analysis of Radial Keratotomy in Human Cadaver Eyes. *Am J Ophthalmol* 92:172, 1981.

17. Waring G, Moffitt S, Gelender H, Laibson P, Lindstrom R, Myers W, Obstbaum S, Rowsey J, Safir A, Schanzlin D, Bourque J: Rationale for and Design of the National Eye Institute Prospective Evaluation of Radial Keratotomy (PERK) Study. *Ophthalmol* 90:40, 1983.

18. Arrowsmith P, Sanders D, Marks R: Visual, Refractive and Keratometric Results of Radial Keratotomy. *Arch Ophthalmol* 101:873, 1983.

19. Kremer F, Marks R: Radial Keratotomy: Prospective evaluation of safety and efficacy. *Ophthal Surg* 14:925, 1983.

20. Kramer S, Yavitz E, Sene K: Precision Standardization of Radial Keratotomy. *Ophthal Surg* 12:561, 1981.

21. McIntyre D: A New Instrument for Precise Radial Keratotomy. *In* RA Schachar, NS Levy, L Schachar (eds), Keratorefraction. Denison, TX: LAL Publishing, 1980. p 189.

22. Gelender H, Parel J: Vacuum Fixation Ring for Radial Keratotomy. *Ophthal Surg* 15:126, 1984.

23. Unterman S Rowsey J: Diamond Knife Corneal Incisions. *Ophthal Surg* 15:199, 1984.

24. Binder P, Stainer G, Akers P, Zavala E, Dev J: Acute Morphologic Features of Radial Keratotomy. *Arch Ophthalmol*, in press, 1983.

25. Akiyama K, Tanaka M, Kanai A, Nakajima A: Problems Arising From Sato's Radial Keratotomy Procedure in Japan. *CLAO J* 10:179, 1984.

26. Hull D, Farkas S, Green K, Laughter L, Elijah R, Bowman K: Radial Keratotomy—Effect on Cornea and Aqueous Humor Physiology in the Rabbit. *Arch Ophthalmol* 101:479, 1983.

27. Yamaguchi T, Asbell P, Ostrick M, Kissling G, Safir A, Kaufman H: Corticosteroid Therapy After Anterior Radial Keratotomy in Primates. *Am J Ophthalmol* 97:215, 1984.

28. Rowsey J, Balyeat H, Rabinovitch B, Burris T, Hays J: *Complications of Radial Keratotomy*. Acta:XXIV International Congress of Ophthalmology, J.B. Lippincott Co., 1983.

29. Salz J: Progressive Endothelial Cell Loss Following Repeat Radial Keratotomy: A case report. *Ophthal Surg* 13:997, 1982.

Chapter 7

Surgical Armamentarium

Spencer P. Thornton, MD, FACS

SURGICAL ARMAMENTARIUM

Basic to successful incisional refractive surgery is the accurate placement of incisions in a predetermined pattern and accurately determined depth. Avoidance of trauma to the globe during fixation and placement of incisions is of utmost importance. Surgical skill and experience are complemented by proper instrumentation. A number of instruments have been designed to achieve this goal. In this chapter we will discuss the basic marking devices, fixation devices, and instruments and devices for measuring the thickness of the cornea and depth of incisions.

Pre- and Intraoperative Measurement of Corneal Thickness

Accurate measurement of corneal thickness is a prime concern for the refractive surgeon. The precision of the corneal incisions of radial keratotomy requires a degree of accuracy not demanded by any previous form of therapy. For this reason, the trend among refractive surgeons has been to depend on ultrasonic pachymeters with multiple point measurements over the cornea to determine the thickness over the entire cornea rather than just at the center. Many surgeons depend on preoperative pachymetry for determining incision depth. A few do this measurement in the operating room.

The ideal pachymeter should offer accurate and reproducible measurements regardless of the technician-operator. It should be easy to operate in the office or operating room and not require constant attention (such as repeated refilling of the probe tip or having to have a second technician to determine alignment of the probe) and it should not require a second person to record the measurements.

Studies of pachymeters both in the laboratory and in a clinical setting[1,2] have shown that ultrasonic pachymeters generally have high reproducibility, little interobserver variation, and no observer bias in measuring the thickness of either the right or the left cornea. Thus ultrasound is generally more usable than optical pachymetry.

Pachymeters currently available are the Kremer Corneometer, the Corneomap 4500, the Cilco 55 Villaseñor, the Coopervision Pachymeter, the Jedmed Pachysonic II, the Storz CS 1000, and the DGH 1000. Most of these instruments appear to be accurate and reliable but they vary greatly in their ease of operation.[3]

The convenience of a preprogrammed pattern of readings with printouts is shared by the Corneomap 4500, Corneometer, Storz CS 1000, Jedmed Pachysonic, and the DGH 1000. The DGH 1000 has the ability to program any number of readings in any pattern desired. The printer then automatically prints a cross-section picture of the cornea in each meridian with each point identified. A feature available in most units with printers is the predetermined percentage depth, based on surgical requirements, printed out by location. This eliminates the need for manual charting and provides the physician with a permanent record.

Depth Measuring Devices

Intraoperative methods of measuring incision depths are somewhat limited at the present time. Laser interferometry and micro-tipped ultrasonic probes may solve this problem. These are currently in the development stage. Several surgical depth gauges for intraoperative measurement of the depth of incisions have been designed by Shepard, Neumann, Deitz, and others (Figures 7-1, 7-2, and 7-3). These gauges ("dipstick" or "hockey stick" type) are designed to be inserted into the incision and observed under the microscope prior to irrigation at the end of the procedure. They give only an approximation of the depth, however, and therefore are of limited value. Accurate pachymetry and precise setting of the blade length is far more important to determining the depths of incisions. If the surgeon is trying to get down to Descemet's membrane (i.e. maximal depth), visual inspection is necessary, and Bores has designed an incision spreader for this purpose (Figure 7-3). Generally it is not necessary to open the incision for examination. The incision depth and length can be clinically estimated with either the round-tipped Shepard radial keratotomy incision irrigating cannula or the Rainin spatulated-tipped irrigating cannula (Figures 7-4 and 7-5). Presently available depth gauges are better suited for judging the overall continuity of the incision rather than the actual incision depth.

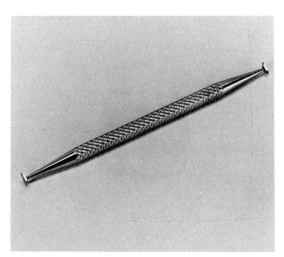

Figure 7-1. Shepard Depth Gauge

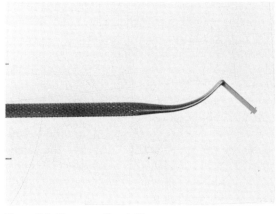

Figure 7-2. Neumann Depth Gauge.

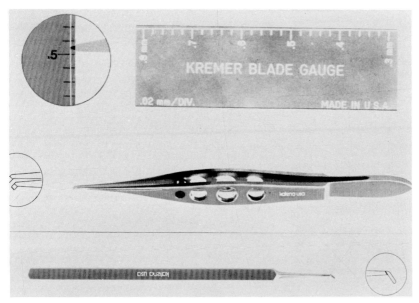

Figure 7-3. Kremer Blade Gauge (top); Bores Incision Spreader (middle); Deitz "hockey stick" Depth Gauge (bottom).

Optical Center Markers

Properly identifying and marking the center of the visual axis is the most important step in the preparation of the eye for surgery. If the optically clear zone is only slightly decentered, the end of the radial incisions may encroach on the visual axis and increase the potential for postoperative problems with glare.

The visual axis of the eye must be determined prior to placement of the optical zone marker, and this can be accomplished in several ways. The most common method is to monocularly fixate the cornea through one ocular of the microscope or through an ophthalmoscope and mark at the point of the light reflex or center of the pupil with a small-gauged needle producing an epithelial defect. Extreme care must be exercised: if the mark is too deep, a stromal dot opacity will result, possibly producing glare problems. A safer method of marking the cornea is with a sharp-tipped HMS Torrington Skin Scribe (Figures 7-6 A, and B) touched to the center of the cornea leaving a dot of gentian violet on the surface. This dot disappears in a few hours. Any epithelial defect resulting from either method rapidly disappears unless it is placed too deeply.

A simple technique for aligning the eye on the visual axis for marking the center of the cornea is to place a small red or white spot (measuring only 2 mm or 3 mm in diameter) in the center of the binocular microscope objective lens between the two observer tubes (Figure 7-7). When viewing the cornea binocularly, the spot is invisible to the surgeon but can be easily fixated by the patient looking up at the microscope. This should be done with room lights only. With the eye accurately centered under the microscope, the center of the visual axis can be marked binocularly.

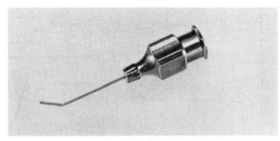

Figure 7-4. Shepard Incision Irrigating Cannula.

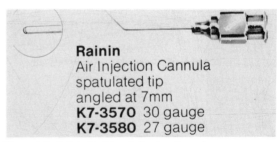

Figure 7-5. Rainin Incision Irrigating Cannula

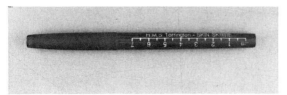

Figure 7-6A. Torrington Gentian Violet Marker (overview).

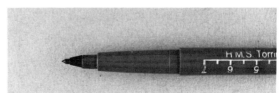

Figure 7-6B. Sharp-tipped Corneal Marker (Close-up view of tip).

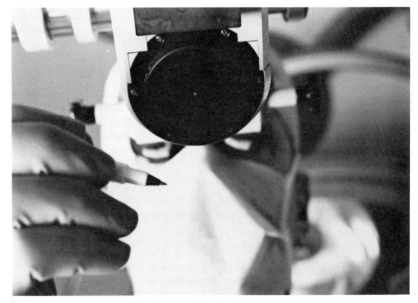

Figure 7-7. Patient's view of fixation spot in center of microscope lens.

Blade Gauges

A variety of blade gauges are available. Their purpose is to verify the setting of blade extension beyond the blade guard or footplate and therefore accuracy is of tantamount importance. Blade gauges should be easy to use under the microscope. The most uncomplicated are those with a continuous line or ramp such as the ones designed by Kremer, Shepard,

Neumann and others (Figures 7-8 and 7-9). These can be used either with metal or gem blades. Several gauges have been designed specifically for the micrometer-handled diamond knives. They have a platform or cradle to protect the tip of the blade and either a linear or "coin" style ramp gauge (Figure 7-10).

Optical Zone Markers

Optical zone markers are designed to be pressed onto the cornea around the optical center mark. These markers—round or oval—usually have a device such as a needle tip or cross hair to indicate the exact center for precise alignment on the cornea. They leave a sharply-defined indentation that disappears in a short time but is visible during the procedure.

The original tube-like optical zone markers of Fyodorov have been redesigned and variously modified by a number of surgeons (Bores, Shepard, Neumann, Hoffer, Kremer, Berkeley, and Thornton) and are available from various instrument companies (Figure 7-11 A, B and C). Few surgeons now use oval optical zone markers as more accurate methods of correcting astigmatism have been developed. But for low degrees of astigmatism, oval optical zone markers are available. The advantage of binocular marking of the optical zone has been achieved by reducing the thickness of the optical zone markers. Optical zone markers only about 1mm high are now available (Storz E-9030 in sizes 3.0 to 5.0 and larger). These overcome the parallax problem found with the thicker optical zone markers and are more easily centered through the binocular microscope.

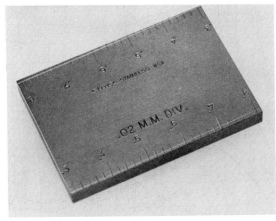

Figure 7-8. Neumann Blade Gauge.

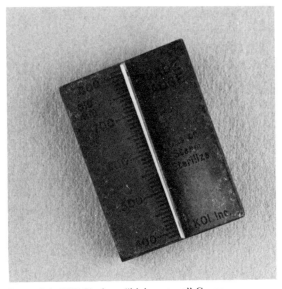

Figure 7-9. KOI Platform "high contrast" Gauge.

Optical zone markers of 6, 7, and 8 mm are also available for accurate delineation of the re-deepening zone for higher power corrections (Figure 7-12).

Radial markers have been found to be an added aid in even distribution of the incisions. This is more important as a greater number of incisions are used. The newer instruments available for marking the radial lines are thinner and less bulky than the original Russian instruments. These have been developed by Bores, Osher, Neumann, Shepard, and others and are available from several instrument manufacturers (Figure 7-13).

Fixation Devices

It is important to immobilize the globe so that the cornea may be cut smoothly by slowly drawing the knife across the cornea in a straight radial manner. When fixated by one point fixation as with most toothed fixation forceps, the eye tends to rotate or wobble as an incision is made, producing a curved or skewed incision (Figures 7-14 and 7-15). The principle of the various fixation forceps which have been designed for globe fixation during radial keratotomy is to prevent torsion of the globe by fixation at more than one point (Figure 7-16). This has been accomplished by various means. Bores, Hofmann, and Kremer have designed U-shaped toothed forceps which grasp the conjunctiva at two points separated by a distance of 3 mm (Bores), 7 mm (Hofmann), or 13 mm (Kremer) (Figure 7-17 A and B). These instruments are available from Katena (Bores, Kremer), Micra (Hofmann) and other companies.

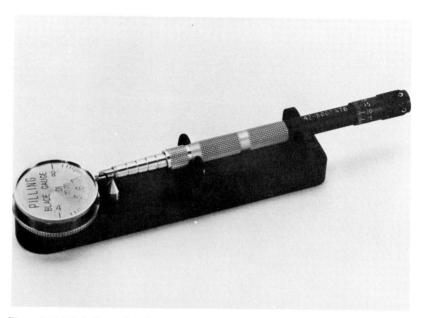

Figure 7-10. "Coin Gauge" and cradle.

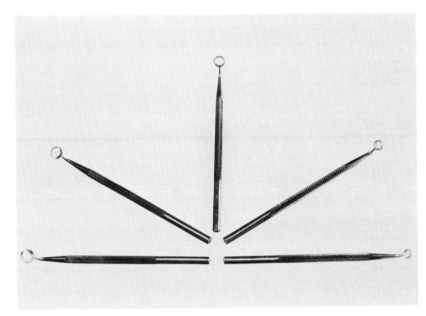

Figure 7-11A. Hoffer "Cross Hair" Optical Zone Markers.

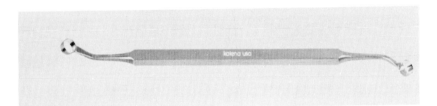

Figure 7-11B. Berkeley Double-ended Markers.

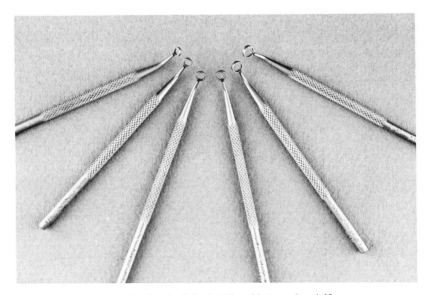

Figure 7-11C. Thornton "Parallax-free" Optical Zone Markers 3 to 4.25 mm.

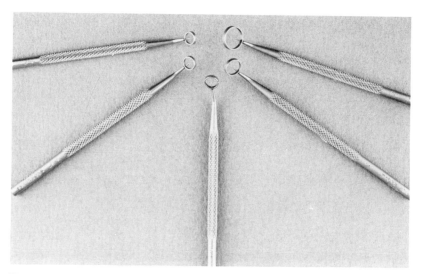

Figure 7-12. Thornton "Parallax-free" Optical Zone Markers 4.5 to 8 mm.

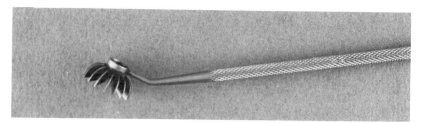

Figure 7-13. Radial Incision Marker.

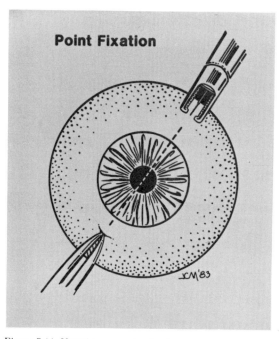

Figure 7-14. Unstable one point fixation.

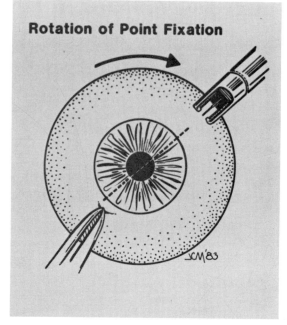

Figure 7-15. Rotation produces skew or curved incision.

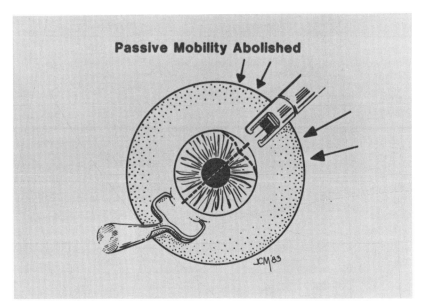

Figure 7-16. Two point fixation reduces rotation.

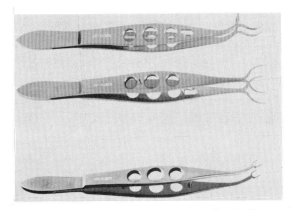

Figure 7-17A. Kremer 13 mm and Bores 3 mm Double Forceps.

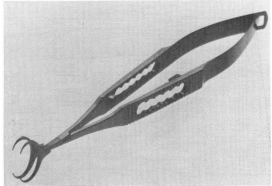

Figure 7-17B. Hofman 7 mm Double Forceps.

A second problem confronts the surgeon after the first two or three incisions are made: not only does the eye tend to rotate but it also begins to soften. It is important that the cornea be as rigid as possible during incision so that the incision may be both straight and equally deep throughout its length. This problem has been solved by the Thornton fixation ring which has 12 atraumatic teeth around a 16 mm ring which is placed around the cornea providing both torsion-free fixation and increased intraocular pressure to assure uniform depth of cuts by simply pressing on the ring as each incision is made. This ring incorporates guide marks on the top of the ring to assist the surgeon in aligning the incisions (Figures 7-18 and 7-19). Another approach to this problem is with the Gelender vacuum fixation ring. Problems frequently encountered with the vacuum ring are conjunctival hemorrhage and postoperative edema. Both instruments allow

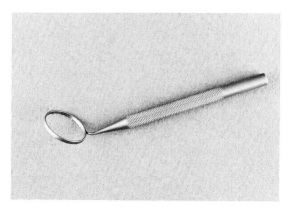

Figure 7-18. Thornton Fixation Ring.

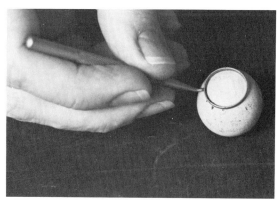

Figure 7-19. Pressure on ring elevates intraocular tension.

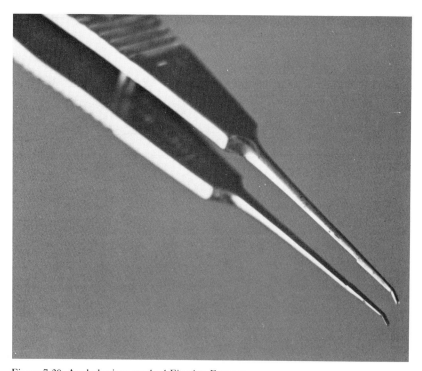

Figure 7-20. Angled micro-toothed Fixation Forceps.

excellent stabilization of the eye during radial keratotomy and provide controllable intraocular pressure elevation with each incision, thereby improving the accuracy for deep reproducible incisions without skew or bevelling.

For those times during the procedure where absolute immobility of the eye is not needed, fixation may be obtained by micro-toothed fixation forceps such as Storz-E 1801 (Figure 7-20). Toothed instruments should be used only on the conjunctiva or sclera; they should never be used on the cornea because of the possibility of epithelial and stromal defects which may delay healing and induce glare. One must beware of instruments that traumatize the cornea or surrounding conjunctiva.

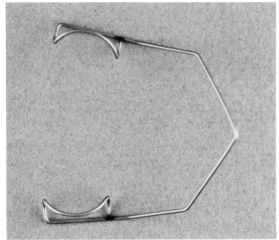

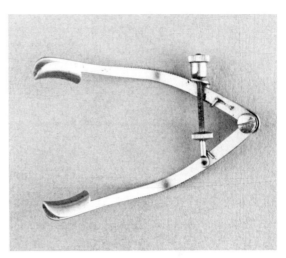

Figure 7-21. Spring Wire Speculum.   Figure 7-22. Blade Speculum.

Irrigation Cannulae

At the conclusion of the keratotomy procedure it is often desirable to wash out the incisions to flush out any blood or cellular debris. This can easily be accomplished with the Shepard radial keratotomy incision irrigating cannula (Storz E-4925, Figure 7-4) or the Rainin cannula (Katena K-73570, Figure 7-5) attached to a 15 cc bottle of balanced salt solution. Gentle irrigation is advised. We do not recommend irrigation with a syringe because of the tendency to flush too forcefully. Sharp-tipped irrigators or pressure in the depth of the incision should be avoided because of the possibility of perforation.

Lid Retraction

Although application of pressure to the globe with a speculum has been advocated to raise the intraocular pressure, this produces inconsistent and unequal pressure with slight but unacceptable distortion of the globe. It is better to have precise control of the pressure as needed. Most refractive surgeons prefer to increase the intraocular pressure as each incision is made with pressure on the fixation ring or forceps.

Any speculum which provides good lid retraction and a clear area to work is satisfactory. A good strong spring wire speculum (Figure 7-21) or a blade speculum (Figure 7-22) is recommended.

Summary

The basic instruments needed for radial keratotomy are optical zone markers from 3 to 5 mm diameters in 0.25 mm increments; optical zone markers of 6, 7, and 8 mm diameters for special applications such as redeepening procedures; radial markers for guiding the incisions; a reliable and easily used fixation device; and a first quality blade and micrometer handle. Steel, diamond, and other blades are covered in Chapter 6. Blade gauges such as the Shepard, Kremer, Neumann, Bores or other similar gauge should always be used to verify the blade length as indicated by the micrometer.

References

1. Thornton SP: A Consumer's Guide to Ultrasonic Pachymeters. American Academy of Ophthalmology, Course 541, Oct 1983.
2. Salz J, Azen SP, Bernstein J, et al.: Evaluation and Comparison of Source of Variability in the Measurement of Corneal Thickness with Ultrasonic and Optical Pachymeters *Ophthal Surg* 14(9):750-754, 1983.
3. Thornton SP: A Guide to Pachymeters *Ophthal Surg* 15(11): 1984.

Chapter 8

Cutting Instruments

Spencer P. Thornton, MD, FACS

CUTTING INSTRUMENTS

In striving for goals of accuracy and predictability the field of bio-engineering has taken on a vital role in ophthalmic surgical technology. Whereas the 1970's brought microsurgery to the fore and we dealt in fractions of a millimeter, with the advent of ultramicrosurgery we're dealing in microns. With these demands for accuracy on a microscopic scale our approach to cutting instruments is more demanding. In this chapter we will look at various cutting instruments and the advantages and disadvantages of each.

Recent Advances

In 1966, reports surfaced about a remarkable new cutting device for eye surgery.[1] The world was served notice that with a diamond blade coupled with a suction ring device, precise, controllable, perfectly-beveled incisions were possible for corneal surgery.[2]

We have now come full circle. Whereas centuries of use and development have assured the steel blade a permanent place in the surgical armamentarium, recent advances in blade technology have pushed the high carbon and stainless steel blades into second place in certain applications.

The chief drawback of the diamond is its cost. Another problem has been shape limitations. With the realization that diamonds could be cut only with certain angles despite their unequaled smoothness and hardness, and could not be reduced to the thinness of steel despite their extreme edge sharpness, manufacturers turned to other gem stones, and ruby and sapphire blades were developed.

No one blade or blade system will satisfy all needs or all surgeons. For some applications, a high carbon steel blade may be desirable. For others a diamond is best. For still other applications, the more recently introduced ruby or sapphire blades may prove advantageous. Though the diamond blade is preferred for the initial incisions of radial keratotomy, the diamond is so smooth that there is virtually no "feel" when Descemet's membrane is incised. The steel blade allows "feel" of tissue and is therefore preferred by some experienced keratorefractive surgeons for peripheral redeepening to prevent repeated perforation.

Steel Versus Diamonds

One recent study[3] compared the incision made by a standard commercially available disposable steel blade and a Micra diamond knife blade in incisions made through calf corneas. With the steel blade (Figure 8-1) the surface epithelium (open arrow) appears irregular and disrupted. The closed arrow points to the underlying stroma, which is smoothly cut but

TABLE 8-1

Origin	Commercial Line	Thickness (inches)	∝ (degrees)
	A. Carbon Steel Alloys		
USSR	Sputnik	0.0033	15
USA	Vxtra	0.0040	14
Japan	Feather	0.0040	12
USA	Gillette Blue Blade	0.0040	14
USA	Clay-Adams	0.0050	17
	B. Stainless Steel		
USA	Vxtra P.S.	0.0040	13
Europe	Wilkinson	0.0040	13
USA	Gillette Super Stainless	0.0040	14
USA	Gillette Platinum Plus	0.0040	12
Europe	Hoffritz	0.0040	13
USA	Schick Plus Platinum	0.0040	15
Europe	Punktal Royal	0.0040	14
USA	Beaver	0.0058	25

TABLE 8-2

Origin	Commercial Line	Hardness (Rc)
	A. Carbon Steel Alloys	
USSR	Sputnik	72.0
USA	Vxtra	70.2
Japan	Feather	68.0
USA	Clay-Adams	66.1
USA	Gillette Super Blue Blade	58.8
USA	Gillette Blue Blade	55.4
	B. Stainless Steel	
USA	Vxtra P.S.	59.4
Europe	Hoffritz	58.7
USA	Gillette Super Stainless	58.0
Europe	Wilkinson	57.2
USA	Gillette Platinum Plus	57.0
USA	Beaver	56.6
Europe	Punktal Royal	56.4
USA	Schick Plus Platinum	55.0

appears to be thrown into a series of folds. With the diamond incision (Figure 8-2) the open arrow indicates the cut epithelium which appears smooth and regular. Individual epithelial cells are seen and appear precisely cut. The incision does not appear to have disrupted this layer. The underlying stroma (closed arrow) appears to be cut sharply with minimal tissue displacement. It should be noted that this comparison was made with a commercially available blade made from an ordinary razor blade. An earlier study[4] was conducted to determine the differences in steel blades available for ophthalmic surgery. To answer the question of which blades pass through tissue more easily a comparison was made of the thickness and angle alpha (angle of the cutting edge) of most available blades (Table 8-1). The hardness, an indication of possible sharpness was also compared (Table 8-2). Steel of the desired hardness for the sharpest surgical blades

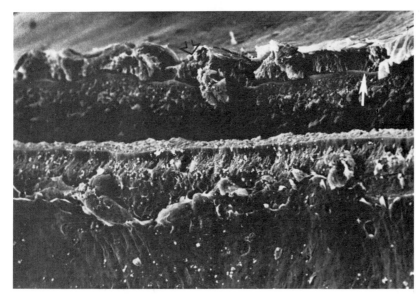

Figure 8-1. Standard razor blade incision (x150).

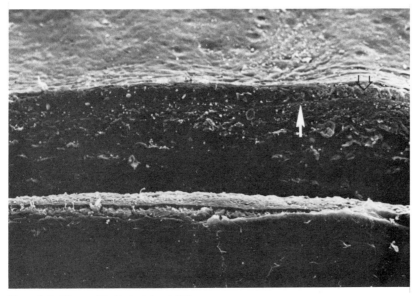

Figure 8-2. Diamond knife incision (x150).

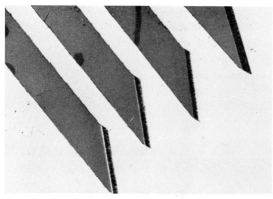

Figure 8-3. Standard razor blade commercially precut for corneal surgery.

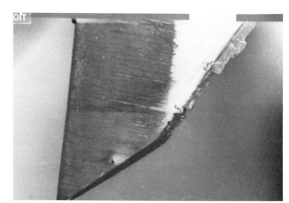

Figure 8-4. Precut RK blade x200 shows poor finishing details.

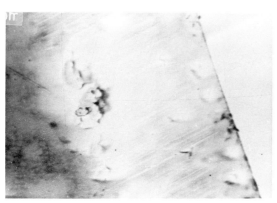

Figure 8-5. The edge of a popular steel blade x200.

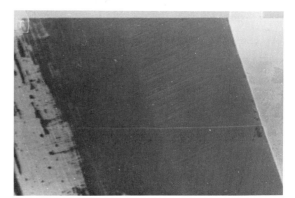

Figure 8-6. Edge of a Vxtra blade x200.

must be made of iron with the highest carbon content possible. Significant differences were found from one manufacturer to another. When an ordinary commercial razor blade is broken or cut into blade fragments for radial keratotomy, quality control has been poor. Figure 8-3 shows four such blades purchased from a major American surgical instrument company. These were sold and represented as being ready for corneal incisions. Even under 20 power magnification round edges and poor finishing are in evidence. When magnification is increased to 200 times (Figure 8-4) rough edges and poor finishing are more evident.

In early studies we wanted to know what made a blade pass smoothly through tissue. What makes a blade stay sharp, and how thin does the blade need to be? In seeking the answers to these questions, significant differences were found between available blades. The ideal blade produces (A) minimal tissue resistance, (B) little tissue displacement, and (C) accurate ability to delineate the incision as to depth and length. Whether cutting from the limbus in, or from the optical zone out, the ideal blade should allow accurate delineation of the central and peripheral ends of the incision.

In seeking the answer to what makes a blade smooth, blade researchers discovered that almost all commercially available razor blades are coated with a material (Dow Corning Vidac or something similar) which prevents rusting and lubricates the blade as used in shaving, but produces drag when pulled *through* tissue.

Only recently have manufacturers realized that ordinary razor blades—however good for shaving—are not adequate for corneal incisions. The finished edge of a typical razor blade (sold as adequate for making blade chips for RK) is illustrated in Figure 8-5. Only two manufacturers produce a blade that is uncoated with highly polished edges necessary for repeated corneal incisions. One of these, Vxtra Corp., is an American company. The excellent edge finish of a Vxtra blade is seen in Figure 8-6.

Though precut RK blades are available, many experienced RK surgeons prefer to make their own blades (Figure 8-7) using a high carbon steel blade and a blade breaker, placing the blade fragment in a micrometer handle

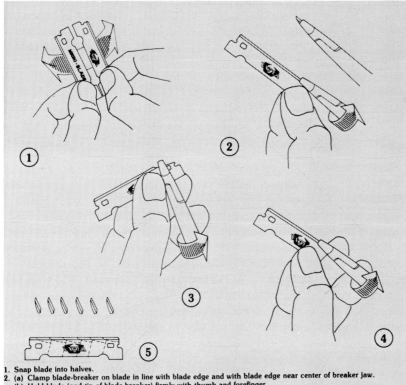

1. Snap blade into halves.
2. (a) Clamp blade-breaker on blade in line with blade edge and with blade edge near center of breaker jaw.
   (b) Hold blade (and tip of blade breaker) firmly with thumb and forefinger.
   (c) Twist blade by rolling breaker. No up or downward movement.
3. Apply breaker across blade below previous break and snap off excess.
4. Repeat steps 2 and 3 for additional blade chips. As many as 10 or 12 microblade chips can be made from each blade. Breaking blades in this manner will give the optimum geometry for R K blades.
   To prevent corrosion of blade edges, wear surgical gloves when handling and breaking blades.
5. Double wrap each blade chip in gas-permeable sterile wrap and gas sterilize.
   Blades prepared in this manner will retain their sharpness indefinitely at room temperature and are immediately ready for use without consuming valuable time in the operating room.

Figure 8-7. Preparing blade chips for RK.

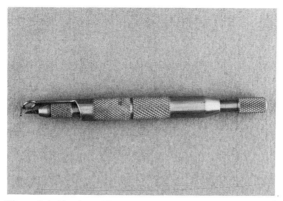

Figure 8-8. Fyodorov Neumann micrometer handle.

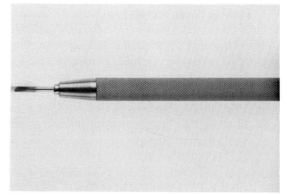

Figure 8-9. Keeler ruby knife.

such as the Neumann modification of the Fyodorov handle (Figure 8-8). The Neumann micrometer handle has a blade guard (footplate) and is designed to allow visualization of the blade in the incision. Because of this blade visibility and the "feel" of the steel blade in tissue, it is preferred by many experienced RK surgeons for peripheral incision redeepening. Free-hand dissections without depth control frequently produce perforations. Experienced RK surgeons limit their free-hand dissections to those occasions where maximal redeepening to Descemet's membrane is needed. Most use an atraumatic incision spreader (see Chapter 7 on Surgical Technique) and a blade with "feel" such as steel or ruby (Figure 8-9).

Diamonds, Sapphires and Rubies

Early diamond knives were advocated for corneal cataract incisions because of their extreme sharpness and absence of drag in tissue.[1] In comparing the edge of a gem quality diamond blade to steel blades a perfect edge sharpness is revealed even at the highest magnification.[5] Figure 8-10 shows the perfect edge of a Micra diamond blade.

Because of the width of early diamond blades corneal tissue was widely separated with the pass of the blade. Diamonds are now available that do not wedge or plow the tissue as the early, wider blades did, and blades as thin as 0.15 mm are available (Figure 8-11). Since a diamond is made of pure carbon atoms in a crystal matrix, its structure allows for a very sharp edge without honing. No pores are present in the diamond, and therefore ultrasonification of the surface between cases allows for easy cleaning. Diamond blades may be flash autoclaved between surgical procedures or gas sterilized.

Diamond blades are now available in many configurations (Figure 8-12) and a recent innovation available from Micra Corp. is a diamond blade with cutting edges on both leading and trailing surfaces for more accurate delineability of the incision length (Figure 8-13).[6] Another gem blade that offers thinness combined with a more desirable cutting edge is the Xtal sapphire blade available from Katena (Figure 8-14).

Currently available diamond knives for radial keratotomy feature

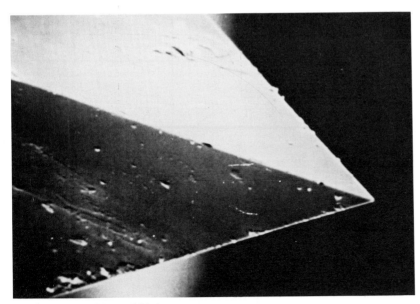

Figure 8-10. Micra Diamond Blade.

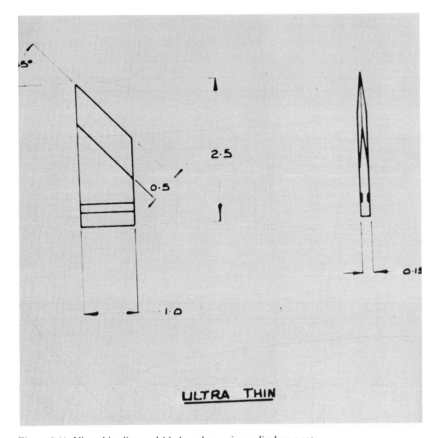

Figure 8-11. Ultra-thin diamond blade reduces tissue displacement.

USE	MODEL	DIAMOND	FOOT
RK	III	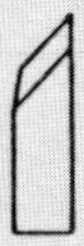 45° Edge	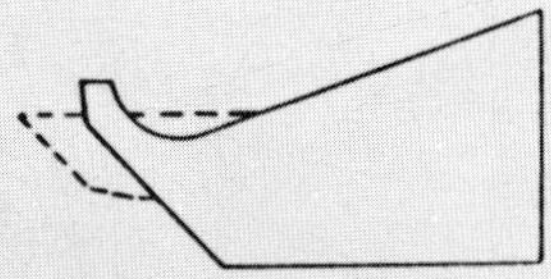
Scleral Resection	Freehand	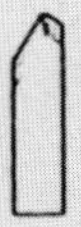 Hex-Facet Edge Tri Edge	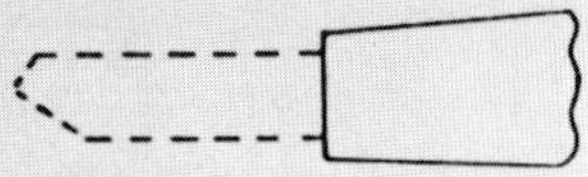
RK	Neumann	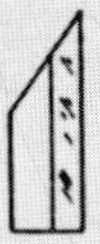 Vertical Edge	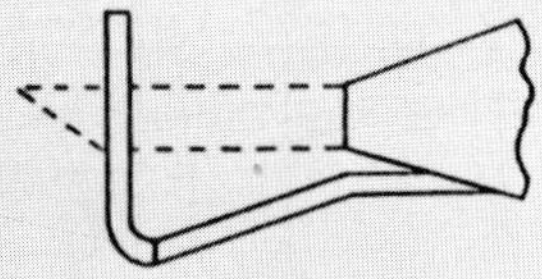
RK	III-V	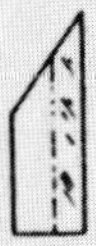 Vertical Edge	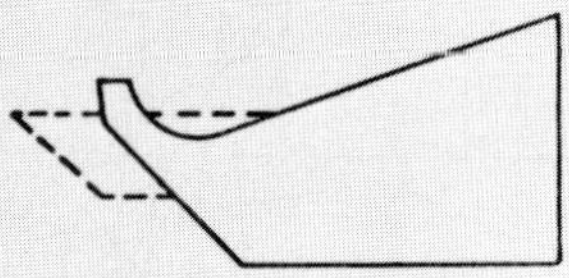
Astigmatism Ruiz	VI	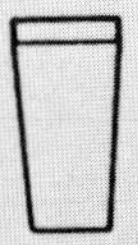 Straight 2.5 mm Edge	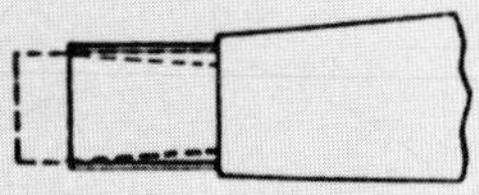
Anterior Chamber	Freehand	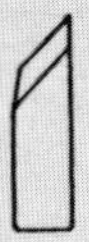 45° Edge	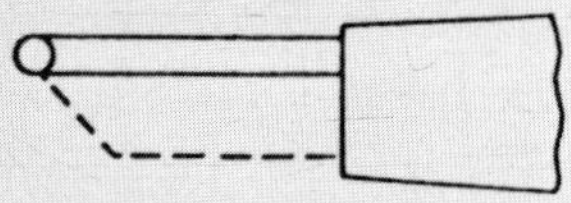
Wedge Resection	MI	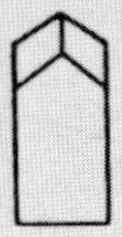 Spear 30°/45° Edge	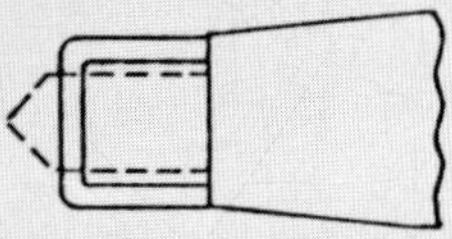

Figure 8-12. Diamond blades, cut to various angles for special uses.

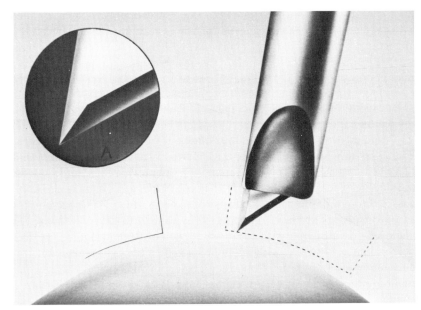

Figure 8-13. Cutting edge on both leading and trailing surfaces.

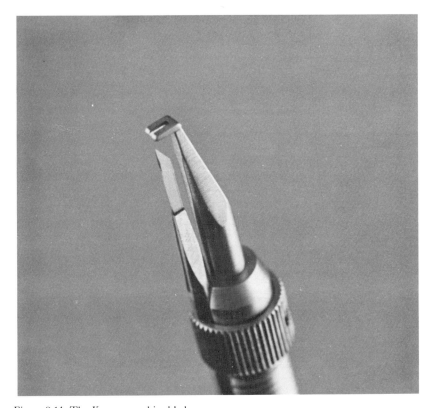

Figure 8-14. The Katena sapphire blade.

micrometer handles with extremely accurate adjustments possible (Figures 8-15, 8-16 and 8-17). Advantages of the titanium handle of the Micra knife are its strength and stability combined with light weight, and its dark surface reduces reflection under the microscope. The easy to adjust micrometer handle of the Pilling Diamond Knife is shown in Figure 8-18.

Though thickness and steep blade angle are advantages, there is some debate as to the advantage of a diamond blade with cutting edges both on the leading and trailing surface. This blade was developed because of the "T" type incision that results at the point of entry of most diamond blades. The ultra-thin diamond blades have partially solved this problem and retain a flat back edge which acts as a "stop" to prevent back cutting. With the double-bladed diamond knife that safety factor is gone, so the knife passes through tissue without resistance in either direction. This requires an extremely steady hand and precise fixation of the eye. With the flat blade guards available with the double-bladed diamond knife a perfect perpendicular entry cut without shelving is possible. Most radial keratotomy surgeons prefer the thin steep-angled diamond blade with a flat trailing edge to cut in one direction only. With the new thinner blade guards, smooth, precise incisions are possible with good visibility of the blade while in the incision (Figure 8-19). Excellent diamond blades and micrometer handles are available from several manufacturers.

Lasers and Other Magic

Of the numerous lasers currently available, several are being used in anterior segment surgery to cut clear or relatively clear tissue such as lens capsules and vitreous strands. The laser appears to offer virtually unlimited

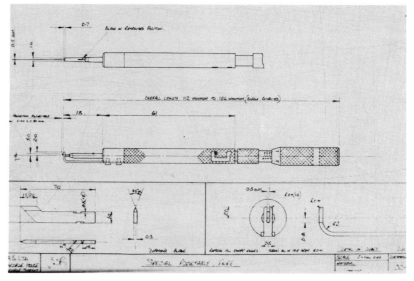

Figure 8-15. Schematic detail of micrometer knife handle.

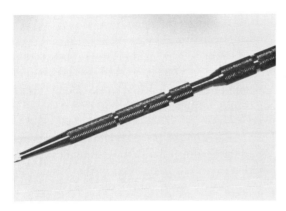

Figure 8-16. The Micra Diamond knife.

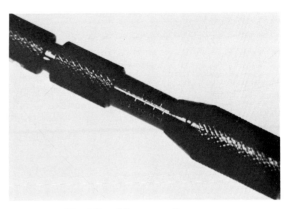

Figure 8-17. The Micra Micrometer Gauge.

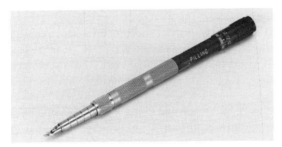

Figure 8-18. Pilling Diamond Blade and Micrometer and Handle.

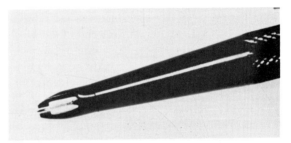

Figure 8-19. This blade guard allows better visibilty of blade in incision.

opportunities for further ocular application. Laser interferometry and micro-tipped ultrasonic probes may be combined with lasers such as the Excimer to cut precise depth incisions into clear cornea. The Excimer laser has the potential of greater precision with less tissue trauma than any knife and does not distort or displace tissue. It can be focused precisely and vaporizes tissue at the cellular level. The clinical applications for incisions such as in radial keratotomy are currently in the development stage. As other laser systems are developed, we will have the capability of delivering energy at differing wavelengths for specific effects and we will have control by microprocessors and fiberoptic cables for direct corneal application.

Care of Gem Blades

Despite best efforts of manufacturers, microscopic particles, stain or other contaminates may be present on blades or in handles provided. All blades and handles should be thoroughly cleaned by soaking or ultrasound, then rinsed with distilled water before sterilization and first use.

The Diamond

The diamond blade is made from a gem quality diamond and is the hardest element known to man. Because of its extremely thin sharp edge it can be damaged easily and should never be touched to any metal surface.

When the diamond blade is passed from assistant to surgeon it should be passed in the blade retracted position.

After the knife is used by the surgeon the blade should be immediately flushed off with sterile distilled water squirted with force through a syringe. Saline may be used if immediately rinsed in distilled water. Never allow blood, tissue or saline solution to dry on the blade as it makes it susceptible to cracking and edge chipping when autoclaved.

If blood or cellular debris has been allowed to dry on the diamond, a Micra diamond knife cleaning block should be used to remove the film from the diamond blade in the following steps. a) Wet one end of the Micra cleaning block with two or three drops of water. b) Extend the diamond blade very carefully, then using a vertical up-and-down motion, pierce the wet end of the block several times. c) Repeat this procedure, piercing the dry side of the block vertically several times.

After extended use a film may be noted on the diamond blade and it can then be cleaned by the following steps. a) Place the knife with the blade retracted in a shallow pan of distilled water with one tablet of enzyme cleaner (Alcon or Allergan soft contact lens enzymatic cleaner) and soak for six to eight hours. b) Clean in ultrasonic bath. c) Rinse with distilled water and repeat the cleaning block procedure as above.

The diamond knife can be sterilized by any conventional method such as gas or steam autoclaving.

The Sapphire

The sapphire blade is made of a crystal sapphire and is extremely sharp and delicate. It requires careful handling. Any contact with metal may chip the gem.

After each use, the blade should be flushed off immediately with sterile distilled water squirted with force through a syringe. Saline may be used if immediately rinsed in distilled water. Never allow blood, tissue or saline solution to dry on the gem as it makes it susceptible to cracking and edge chipping when autoclaved. If a film remains on the gem it may be plunged vertically into a wet sponge such as the Micra diamond knife cleaning block. Never use a dry sponge and never use material which may leave lint on the blade. If a film deposits on the blade and is not cleaned with normal cleaning procedures, it may be soaked in a mild soap solution and then rinsed with distilled water. The Xtal sapphire blade should not be exposed to ultrasonic cleaning.

The sapphire blade and micrometer handle may be sterilized with steam autoclave, ethylene oxide gas or dry heat.

The Ruby

The ruby blade should be stored in its retracted position until the moment of use. Do not wipe or rub the tip. A wiping motion against the blade will dull the cutting edge.

After each use flush the blade off with sterile distilled water squirted with force through a syringe. Saline may be used if immediately rinsed in distilled water. Never allow blood, tissue or saline solution to dry on the blade as it makes it susceptible to cracking and edge chipping when autoclaved.

After every 15 or 20 uses, place the ruby knife (blade retracted in handle) in ultrasonic cleaner and then rinse with distilled water. DO NOT WIPE BLADE.

When a film remains on the blade use the following procedure: a) Place ruby knife (blade retracted) in a shallow pan in distilled water with one tablet of enzyme cleaner (Alcon or Allergan soft contact lens enzymatic cleaner), soak for six to eight hours. b) Clean in ultrasonic cleaner as in step 2 above. c) Rinse with distilled water; do not wipe blade. d) The ruby blade can be sterilized by autoclaving, soaking, gas sterilization or dry heat. Always sterilize with the blade in the retracted position.

Summary

The choice between currently available cutting instruments depends upon the surgeon's experience, philosophy and pocketbook. Disposable steel blades are quite popular and offer convenience, dependability and low cost. Experience has shown however that with precut blades quality control varies from manufacturer to manufacturer. This variability may be critical when the surgery involves the precision required in radial keratotomy. A diamond blade offers unequaled sharpness, reliability and reproducibility. The main drawback of the diamond is its high cost, but this must be considered in the light of its reusability over a long period of time with proper care. Other gem blades such as the sapphire appear to offer a desirable compromise with excellent sharpness, long life and reasonable cost. Regardless of what blade is used, an accurate micrometer handle is essential to provide precise control of blade extension for tolerances in the order of ±5 microns.

References

1. Durham DG: Diamond Knives in Ocular Surgery. *Am J Ophthalmol* 62(1):16-19, 1966.
2. Durham DG and Luntz MH: Diamond Knife in Cataract Surgery, *Br J Ophthalmol* 52(2):206-209, 1968.
3. Galbavy EJ: Use of Diamond Knives in Ocular Surgery. *Ophthal Surg* 15(3):203-205, 1984.
4. Thornton SP: Blade Technology in Radial Keratotomy. *In* Refractive Keratoplasty, Denison, TX: LAL Publ Co, 1983, pp 187-197.
5. Rowsey JJ, Balyeat HD, Yeisley KP: Diamond Knife. *Ophthal Surg* 13(4):279-282, 1982.
6. Yeisley KP: Personal communication with President, Micra Titanium Corp.

Chapter 9

Surgical Technique and Complications

Andrew O. Lewicky, MD, FACS

Photographs of Micra Diamond Instruments are reproduced by permission of Micra Titanium Corp.
Photographs of Vxtra Blades are reproduced by permission of Vxtra Corp.
Photograph of Xtal Sapphire Blade is reproduced by permission of Katena Corp.

SURGICAL TECHNIQUE AND COMPLICATIONS

The basic surgical principles of radial keratotomy have not changed since its inception by Fyodorov in the early 1970s, as first performed in the United States by Bores in 1978, and as subsequently described by Fyodorov and Durnev in the American literature in 1979.[1] Although there have been many modifications and variations of Fyodorov's basic surgical technique, the primary factors responsible for the clinical effect as well as the fundamental technical goals of surgery also have remained the same.

The surgical technique is deceptively simple: create a given number of linear radial incisions at a prescribed depth through the corneal epithelium and stroma while preserving an adequate clear central optical zone. In one way or another all of the surgical modifications have attempted to facilitate this surgical process. The difficulty lies in the ability of the human hand— using instruments of finite sharpness and accuracy—to make consistently straight, 90% uniform depth incisions into biological tissue that measures approximately 500 microns in thickness at the edge of the optical zone and increases in thickness toward the periphery.

Most radial keratotomy surgeons today would agree that the primary factors responsible for the surgical effect of radial keratotomy are size of the optical zone (the smaller the optical zone the greater the effect), depth of the incisions (very deep incisions are required to obtain a lasting effect), and number of incisions (increasing effect with more incisions). Other factors of importance include age of the patient (younger less effect, older more effect), sex of the patient (up to age 40, females less effect than males), intraocular pressure (very low IOPs less effect, ocular hypertensives more effect), and perhaps corneal thickness (thick corneas more effect). Factors which affect predictability of radial keratotomy are covered in greater detail in Chapter 5.

Anesthesia for Radial Keratotomy Surgery

Radial keratotomy surgery can be performed under general anesthesia, local retrobulbar anesthesia/akinesia with intravenous sedation, or topical anesthesia with or without intravenous sedation. The type of anesthesia utilized is dependent on the patient and surgeon preference. Although the risks of general anesthesia in the typical young or middle-aged healthy radial keratotomy patient are minimal, most surgeons utilize general anesthesia only in isolated instances of highly anxious patients who demand it.

Retrobulbar injection is utilized by a decreasing number of surgeons. Although it is not without risk (one known blind eye from perforation of the globe by the retrobulbar needle[2]), retrobulbar injection has several advantages: deeper and prolonged anesthetic effect (if bupivacaine used) resulting in increased patient comfort during surgery and the first 24 hours after surgery, extraocular muscle akinesia resulting in greater control of the position of the eye during surgery, and ability to use certain fixation devices (suction rings) to both fixate the eye and increase intraocular pressure during surgery.

Most radial keratotomy surgeons, however, use topical anesthesia (either tetracaine, lidocaine, or proparacaine) with or without intravenous sedation. The primary reasons for the widespread use of topical anesthesia are safety and simplicity. If the procedure is performed without intravenous sedation, attendance of an anesthesiologist is not necessary and the cost to the patient is decreased. The surgeon can greatly reduce the patient's anxiety by calmly describing each step of the preparation routine to the patient, explaining what to anticipate as the drape is applied, the lid speculum is inserted, eye drops are instilled, level of anesthesia of perilimbal conjunctiva is tested, and the fixation forceps is applied to begin the surgery. Disadvantages of topical anesthesia include increased patient awareness resulting in some degree of blepharospasm and Bell's phenomenon. Although topical anesthesia easily eliminates corneal sensations, achieving adequate perilimbal conjunctival anesthesia may require numerous applications of the topical anesthetic in the anxious patient. In addition, extraocular muscle resistance to the surgeon's attempted rotation of the globe as well as "involuntary" attempts by the patient to move his eye may occur with topical anesthesia. Intravenous sedation decreases and, in some cases, eliminates many of these difficulties.

Preoperative Patient Preparation

In the Office. Each radial keratotomy patient must receive a detailed ophthalmic examination, consultation, and informed consent document to sign. The consent form should list the goals of surgery, describe alternatives to surgery, and explain known risks and complications. The patient should study and sign the informed consent document prior to the day of surgery. Informed consent is extremely important. It should clearly identify the visual goals of the individual patient in seeking keratotomy surgery, assess the statistical probability of the surgery achieving these goals, and finally document the patient's understanding of the surgical goals and willingness to undergo the surgery in an attempt to achieve these visual goals. This subject is explored further in Chapter

In the Preoperative Hold Area. The systemic preoperative medications used vary depending upon whether general or local anesthesia is utilized. For topical anesthesia, oral diazepam 10 mg on call is usually sufficient, providing enough sedation to relieve minor anxiety yet maintaining enough alertness to allow for good patient cooperation. In addition, a nonsteroidal anti-inflammatory drug such as fenoprofen has been useful in decreasing postoperative lid and conjunctival edema, resulting in greater patient comfort. This medication is started as a single preoperative dose of oral fenoprofen 300 mg on call and continued postoperatively for one week with 300 mg given three times per day after meals unless signs of gastrointestinal intolerance develop.

When Bores first introduced radial keratotomy surgery in the United States, he recommended dilating the pupil before surgery in order to better visualize the incisions against the red reflex. However, this practice is now limited to cases of reoperation which require additional incisions, primarily in patients with lightly colored blue irides. As a result, most surgeons either use nothing topically or very weak strength pilocarpine to constrict the pupil (pilocarpine 1%, 2 drops on call). A constricted pupil decreases the patient's sensitivity to the light of the operating microscope, increases the ease and accuracy of marking the visual axis, and decreases Bell's phenomenon during the course of surgery.

In the Operating Room. Prior to the preparation and draping, the position of the patient's head, the operating microscope, and the surgeon's hands should be checked. The patient's head may be secured with tape to the operating table to insure immobilization and proper position with the plane of the iris in a horizontal orientation. The body of the operating microscope is then positioned perpendicular to this plane, forming as close to a 90° angle as possible (Figure 9-1). Two drops of a topical anesthetic (e.g. proparacaine 0.5% or tetracaine 0.5%) are instilled in each eye and a metal or plastic shield is taped over the fellow eye. The combination of the topical anesthetic and protective shield makes it easier for the patient to keep both eyes open during surgery, reducing the Bell's phenomenon tendency. The protective shield also allows the surgeon to rest his wrist over this area without causing patient discomfort. A plastic air cannula is taped to the

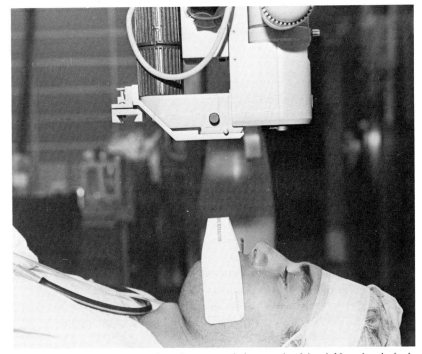

Figure 9-1. Position of the operating microscope relative to patient's head. Note that the body of the microscope is perpendicular to the patient's iris plane.

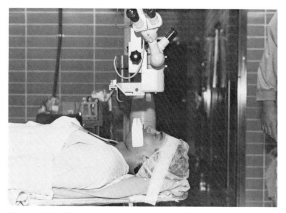

Figure 9-2A. Patient's head with metal shield over fellow eye (not shown), drape retractor, and air cannula in place just prior to draping. Note tape securing forehead to surgical table.

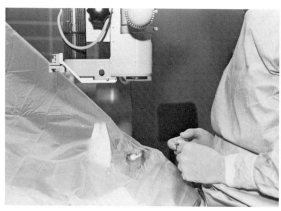

Figure 9-2B. Same patient as in Figure 9-2A after plastic drape and lid speculum are in place.

patient's face and the surgical area is prepped with povidone-iodine solution and dried. A disposable drape retractor is applied (Figure 9-2). The patient's head is now draped with a disposable plastic incise drape. The surgeon should check his hand position for comfort and stability. Arm-rests can be used if so desired to enhance the surgeon's steadiness. However, bracing one's wrists on the patient's head is preferable since this method assures that the surgeon's hands will move together with any unanticipated movement of the patient's head (Figure 9-3).

Basic Radial Keratotomy Operative Technique

The following description details the surgical technique employed by the author at the present time. Other approaches are discussed under "Variations" within each subsection of this chapter.

Marking Visual Axis and Optical Zone. After the patient is draped, two drops of the topical anesthetic are instilled and a solid-blade wire self-retaining lid speculum is inserted. The 12 o'clock and 6 o'clock limbal conjunctiva are marked with a skin marking pencil to define the 90° meridian (Figure 9-4). These reference marks help ensure accurate orientation of both the radial incisions and any astigmatism-reducing incisions. The intensity of the coaxial light source of the OpMi-6 microscope is decreased by interposing the green filter. If electrical engineering support is available, a rheostat can be installed which will control the intensity of the coaxial light, and makes the use of the green filter unnecessary.

The patient is asked to fixate on the center of the filament of the coaxial light, the reflection of which is visualized by the surgeon monocularly on the surface of the cornea (Figure 9-5). The visual axis is marked with a fine blunt-tipped instrument such as a 0.2 mm lens manipulator (some use a needle point) by making a dimpled impression on the corneal surface

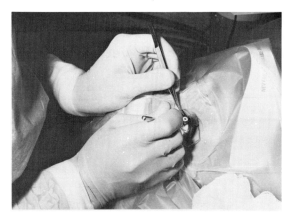

Figure 9-3. Surgeon's wrists braced on patient's forehead.

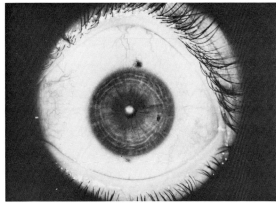

Figure 9-4. The 12 o'clock and 6 o'clock limbal conjunctival marked with dye to identify the 90° meridian.

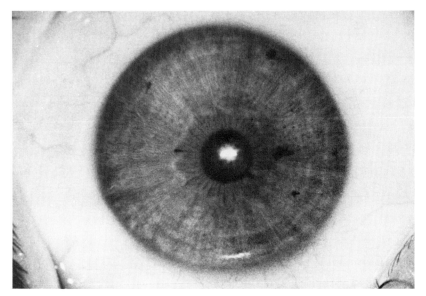

Figure 9-5. Corneal light reflex from coaxial light on Op-Mi 6 Zeiss Microscope.

approximately 0.3 mm inferior to the opposite end of the reflection of the filament on the corneal surface, ie, left end of reflex if surgeon is viewing with right eye (Figure 9-6). The patient is then asked to look away for a second and then re-fixate on the filament to verify correct placement of the dimple on the visual axis. The appropriate size optical zone marker is centered on the visual axis dimple and the optical zone is firmly marked while the eye is fixated with two point fixation forceps (Figure 9-7). If the case requires redeepening of the incisions, a second larger optical zone is marked (5 mm or 6 mm) with a second marker or with a concentric 3/5 mm marker (Figure 9-8). In some cases a third zone can be marked using a combination 3/5/7 mm marker. If general anesthesia is used, the visual axis is marked prior to the induction of anesthesia and draping.

Variations: Marking Visual Axis and Optical Zone. The visual axis can be marked very accurately using a monocular ophthalmoscope (Figure

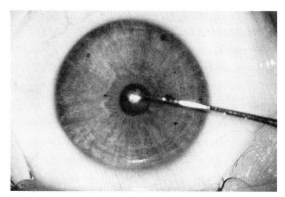

Figure 9-6A. Beginning of the visual axis marking sequence using corneal light reflex from coaxial light of Op-Mi 6 Zeiss microscope. Note that the tip of the marking instrument is just below (to compensate for the 7° displacement of the light by the Zeiss microscope) and to the left of center of the corneal light reflex (surgeon is marking visual axis with his right eye).

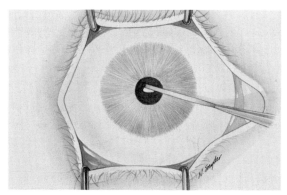

Figure 9-6B. Diagram of Figure 9-6A.

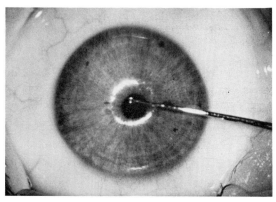

Figure 9-6C. Corneal surface being marked with a fine blunt-tipped instrument (lens manipulator). Note circular reflex indicating extent of indentation.

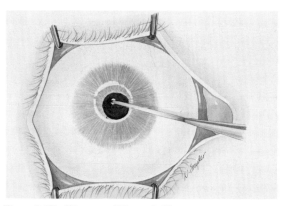

Figure 9-6D. Diagram of Figure 9-6D.

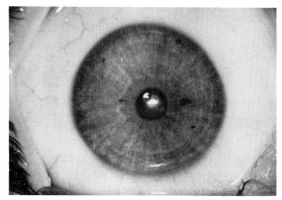

Figure 9-6E. Resultant dimple on corneal surface. Apparent decentration due to angle kappa and camera view through beam splitter. Patient should be asked to look away and then refixate on the microscope light to verify correct placement of the visual axis mark.

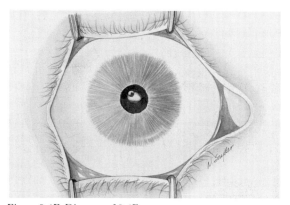

Figure 9-6F. Diagram of 9-6E.

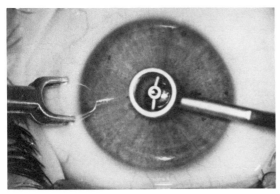

Figure 9-7A. Circular sight marker is centered on the dimple. Note tiny reflection within marker circular sight.

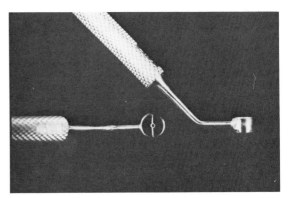

Figure 9-7B. Circular sight optical zone markers, two views.

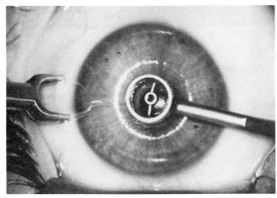

Figure 9-7C. Marking optical axis. Note extent of corneal indentation by circular reflex.

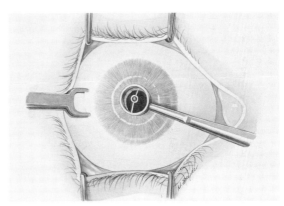

Figure 9-7D. Diagram of 9-7C.

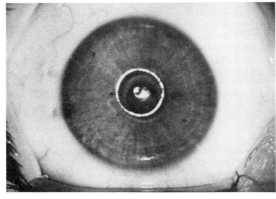

Figure 9-7E. Resultant optical axis mark on corneal surface.

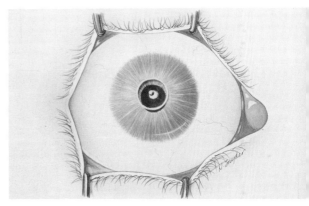

Figure 9-7F. Diagram of Figure 9-7E.

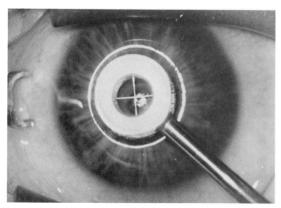

Figure 9-8A. Marking two optical zones with Kremer 3/5 mm marker.

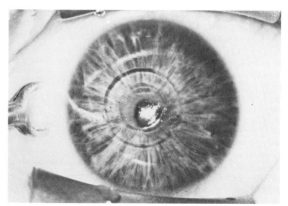

Figure 9-8B. Concentric 3/5 mm optical axis marks resulting from procedure in Figure 9-8A.

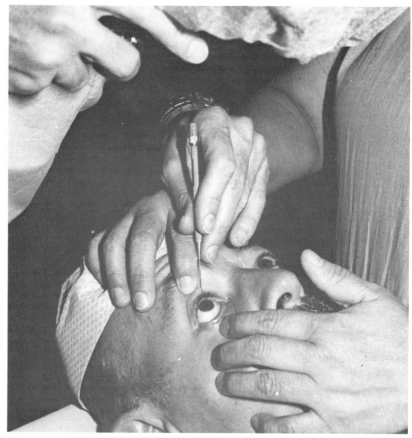

Figure 9-9. Marking the visual axis with a direct ophthalmoscope.

9-9). The smallest light aperture of the ophthalmoscope is chosen with a +3.00 viewing lens on the dial. The patient's fellow eye is patched and he is asked to fixate on this light with the operative eye. The surgeon then marks the visual axis in similar fashion by making a mark on the corneal surface corresponding to the corneal light reflection. No compensatory displacements are necessary. Although this simple method is very accurate, it does represent an extra preoperative step. The epithelial mark may fade and be hard to find unless stained with fluorescein. If microscopic coaxial illumination is not available, this method of marking the visual axis is very useful.

Another method of marking the visual axis involves the use of the Osher device (Figure 9-10). This apparatus is attached to the operating microscope and channels the coaxial illumination light through a fiberoptic bundle that is aligned perfectly with the surgeon's viewing angle. As the patient fixates on this light the resulting corneal light reflex represents the true visual axis. The only drawback of this device is the low illumination level of the light transmitted through the fiberoptic bundle which results in a very dim, hard to visualize corneal light reflex.

The Polaroid photograph of a corneascope can also be used to determine the position of the visual axis.[3] Here the distance from the visual axis to the nasal limbus (CL) and the horizontal limbus to limbus distance (LL) are measured with calipers on the photograph. The fraction obtained by dividing CL by LL is then used to multiply the patient's actual horizontal limbus to limbus distance as measured in millimeters at surgery with calipers. The resulting product represents an objective distance measurement of the visual center from the nasal limbus.

Villaseñor has devised an opaque 12 mm contact lens with a 200 micron opening positioned just off center. This contact lens is then rotated until the patient can fixate on the coaxial light of the operating microscope through the 200 micron opening. The visual axis is then marked with a blunt needle through this same opening. The main purpose of this contact lens approach is to increase the accuracy of marking the visual center by decreasing the patient's photophobia.

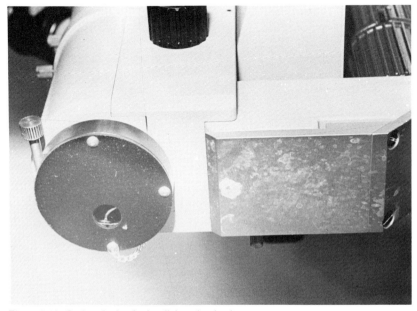

Figure 9-10. Oscher device for localizing visual axis.

Some surgeons omit marking the visual axis as a separate step in the surgical technique. Instead, the corneal light reflex is used as a reference point to mark the optical zone directly with the appropriate size zone marker. This approach saves time. The advantage of marking the visual axis first with a small epithelial defect or dimple is primarily related to the ability to make another small mark if the first did not accurately represent the visual axis. When the visual axis is marked directly with the optical zone marker and then found to be inaccurate, remarking it will result in two circle imprints on the cornea that can lead to confusion during the cutting process (Figure 9-11). Certain surgeons will stain the optical zone marker before use to leave a more easily visible mark on the cornea even when the corneal surface is wet. If a vital stain (such as kitton green or gentian violet) is used, the marker should be applied to a relatively dry corneal surface since a wet surface will not take up the stain as effectively. Other surgeons use fluorescein. If so desired, the corneal surface may be marked with a six- or eight-incision marker aligned (Figure 9-12) with respect to the previously marked 90° meridian conjunctival stains. The six-incision marker can be used for six- and 12-incision cases while the eight-incision marker can be used for four-, eight-, and 16-incision cases.

Complications: Incorrect Marking of Visual Axis. Incorrect marking of the visual axis can produce more glare from incisions that encroach upon the central clear zone. This is particularly important with small optical zone cases (3.0 mm). Large angle kappa patients can produce uncertainty during surgery. The surgeon must develop confidence in his technique of marking the visual axis and not be intimidated by a large positive angle kappa. Prevention in the case of incorrect visual axis is the only solution to avoiding this problem. Hence, the advantage of premarking the visual axis before marking the optical zone.

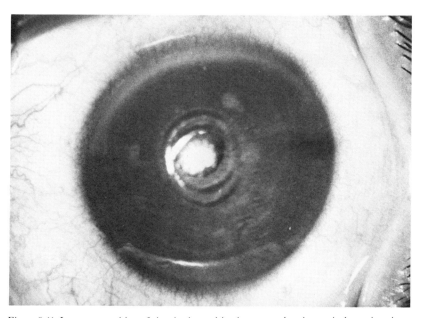

Figure 9-11. Incorrect marking of visual axis resulting in two overlapping optical zone imprints.

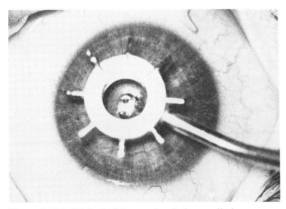

Figure 9-12A. Eight-incision marker being applied to cornea. Note central corneal dimple marking visual axis.

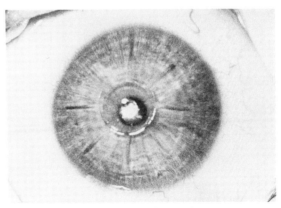

Figure 9-12B. Resultant corneal indentations.

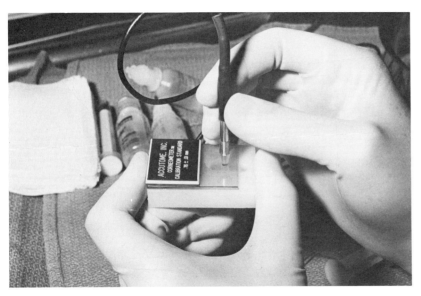

Figure 9-13. Verifying accuracy of ultrasonic probe on test block.

Intraoperative Measurement of Corneal Thickness. After

the patient is draped but prior to insertion of the lid speculum and marking of the visual axis and optical zone, the ultrasonic pachymeter (e.g. Accutome) is prepared, and the sterile probe's accuracy is verified on the test block (Figure 9-13). Following this, the lid speculum is inserted and the visual and optical axes are marked as previously described. The cornea is irrigated with balanced salt solution to insure normal hydration. The sterile probe of the ultrasonic pachymeter under microscopic control is placed over the visual axis and the corneal thickness is recorded. Next the optical zone marker imprint on the corneal surface (easier to see if a dye was used) is straddled by the pachymeter probe and the corneal thickness is measured and recorded in the 12, 3, 6, and 9 o'clock meridians (Figure 9-14). If a second or third zone is to be cut, these same cardinal meridians are measured at the 5 mm and 7 mm zone marks respectively.

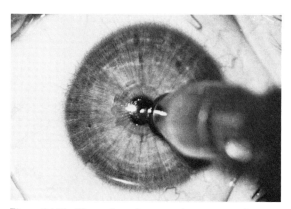

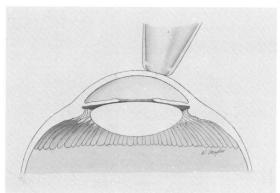

Figure 9-14A. Ultrasonic probe measuring paracentral corneal thickness by straddling visual axis mark on corneal surface. The probe should be kept as normal to the corneal surface as possible.

Figure 9-14B. Diagram of Figure 9-14A. Note optical zone indentation is straddled by ultrasonic probe.

Variations: Pachymetry Measurements. Intraoperative ultrasonic pachymetry is not universally used. The primary advantage of intraoperative ultrasonic pachymetry is the ability to precisely measure the corneal thickness at the exact point where the radial incisions will be started and, in some cases, deepened. This information would appear to offer the surgeon the best chance of achieving deep incisions with the least risk of perforation. Whether or not this high degree of topographical and temporal accuracy is necessary for clinical success is controversial. Disadvantages of intraoperative pachymetry include equipment failure resulting in cancellation of the surgery, prolonged operative time due to the measurements and intraoperative setting of the micrometer knife, and possible epithelial trauma from the transducer tip.

Alternatives include preoperative optical Haag-Streit, optical specular photographic, and ultrasonic pachymetry. There is little doubt that the ultrasonic pachymeter is the most accurate objective method.[4] Whether the corneal thickness readings are performed before surgery in the office or intraoperatively depends on the particular surgical technique used and the ability to obtain accurate office pachymetry readings. Some surgeons feel a central pachymetry reading is sufficient to use as the basis for setting the depth of cut and they use the same formula regardless of the size of the optical zone. Others utilize the central reading as the basis for an extrapolation formula for various optical zones, adding an incremental amount to the central reading.

Setting Micrometer Diamond Knife. After the pachymetry readings are obtained, the lid speculum is removed while the micrometer diamond knife is prepared in order to prevent corneal thinning from dehydration (cornea may thin as much as 10% in 10 minutes).[5] The thinnest paracentral pachymeter reading is selected and used as a guide for setting the micrometer diamond knife. The accuracy of the micrometer setting is verified on a blade gauge specifically designed for that particular diamond knife and incorporates a cradle-type holder that secures the knife and prevents damage to the diamond tip (Figure 9-15). The surgeon must align the gauge properly by sighting with one eye, making sure the side against which the bladeguard of the knife rests is perfectly vertically in line with the surgeon's visual axis through the microscope. If a second zone is to be incised, a second knife is set to the appropriate second zone depth. If preoperative pachymetry is used, the knife blade(s) is(are) set before starting the case.

Making the Corneal Incisions.

The lid speculum is reinserted. Additional topical anesthetic drops are instilled as necessary, depending on the sensitivity of the perilimbal conjunctiva. The patient is informed that there may be a pressure sensation during the cutting process and that the patient should not resist any rotation movement of the eye made by the surgeon but should simply allow his eye to be moved easily. The conjunctival fornices are thoroughly dried and the corneal surface at the optical

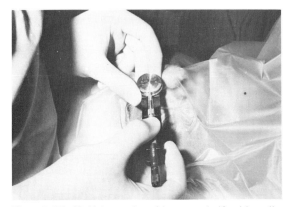

Figure 9-15A. Verifying setting of Accutome knife with cradle-blade gauge.

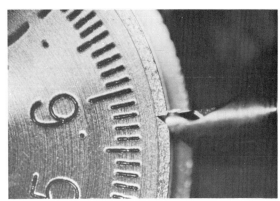

Figure 9-15B. Close-up view of coin-gauge and diamond blade tip.

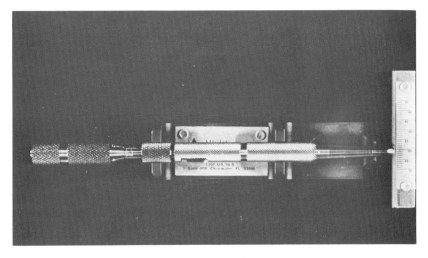

Figure 9-15C. Micra diamond knife with cradle-blade gauge.

zone is dried with a microsponge just enough to reveal the previously made indentation (Figure 9-16). (Muro-cel sponges may leave less particulate material than Weck-cel sponges.) The knife blade and guard have likewise been previously dried with a microsponge if necessary. Although a very slight amount of epithelial moisture is desirable to act as a lubricant between the knife guard and the epithelial surface, it is important to be sure that no excess fluid is trapped within the knife mechanism and shaft (Figure 9-17) or in the conjunctival fornices. The later appearance of fluid from these sources may either mask or simulate a corneal perforation. The assistant or scrub nurse can be instructed to keep the tip of a microsponge visible within the microscope's objective field to allow the surgeon quick access for drying the knife tip and guard if fluid should appear.

The first incision is made in the nasal horizontal meridian. The horizontal incisions are the easiest to perform and the nasal cornea is thicker than the temporal cornea. For the right eye, the fixation forceps is held in the right hand fixing the eye in the 9 o'clock meridian while the knife is held in the left hand. The mechanics of performing an individual incision can be divided into four steps:

1) Fixation and rotation of the eye to the proper starting point.
2) Perpendicular plunging of the knife at the optical zone boundary line.
3) Lateral cutting of the incision.
4) Termination of the incision.

1) The temporal perilimbal conjunctiva and Tenon's capsule are grasped and the eye rotated slightly medially if necessary to position the optical zone boundary line directly underneath the tip of the knife. The knife is held in a position normal to the corneal surface (Figure 9-18).

2) The tip of the blade enters at the inside edge of the optical zone mark. The knife is plunged firmly in this perpendicular position slightly indenting the cornea to insure a deep entry (Figure 9-19). The knife is maintained in this position for about two seconds to effect deep penetration of the blade tip and a right-angle incision profile at the edge of the optical zone. In

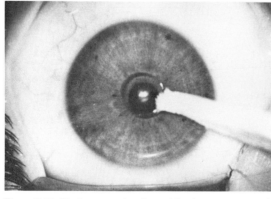

Figure 9-16. Drying corneal surface with microsponge, revealing previously placed optical zone indentation.

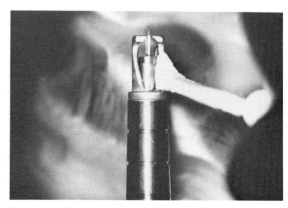

Figure 9-17. Drying knife blade and guard with microsponge.

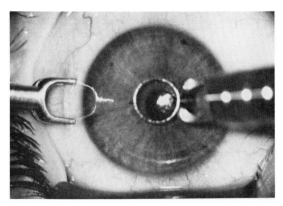

Figure 9-18A. Starting position for first incision. Knife is held normal to the corneal surface with blade tip at the inside edge of the corneal optical zone indentation mark.

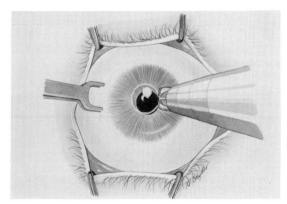

Figure 9-18B. Diagram of Figure 9-18A.

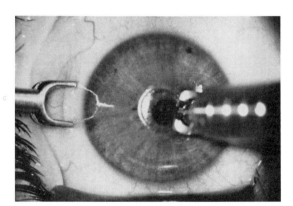

Figure 9-19A.

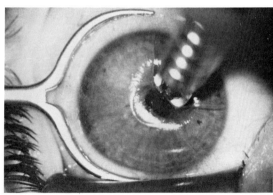

Figure 9-19B.

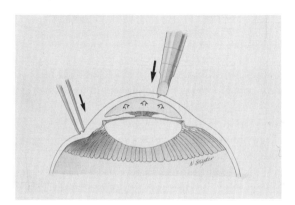

Figure 9-19C.

Figure 9-19A. Plunging knife blade at the optical zone. Note corneal surface distortion due to downward pressure by knife.

Figure 9-19B. Another example of initial plunge phase. Note perpendicularity of knife and circular corneal reflex indicating firm downward pressure.

Figure 9-19C. Diagram of Figures 9-19A and B. Note arrows indicating downward pressure by both knife and the fixation forceps in order to increase intraocular pressure insuring deep corneal penetration to full length of blade extention.

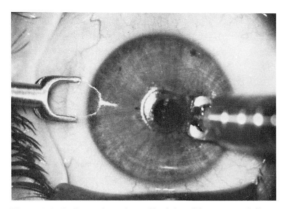

Figure 9-20A. Lateral cutting of incision. Note corneal distortion indicating extent of downward pressure by knife.

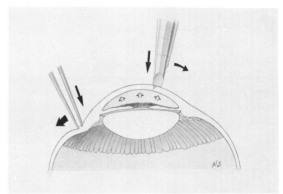

Figure 9-20B. Diagram showing relatively more rotation by forceps while knife is held normal to corneal surface and moved as necessary. Note continued downward pressure by fixation forceps to maintain globe firmness.

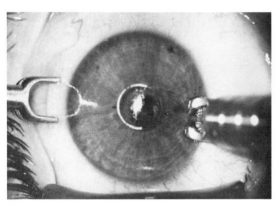

Figure 9-21A. Approaching end of first radial incision. Note continued corneal surface distortion due to downward pressure by knife.

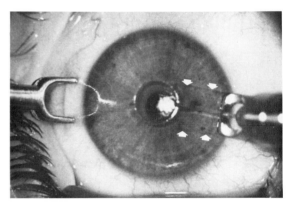

Figure 9-21B. Termination point of incision 0.5 mm from limbus. Note excellent view of limbal area through blade guard of Accutome knife. Also note corneal epithelium indentation (arrows) from blade guard indicating degree of downward pressure exerted during the cutting sequence.

the rare event that a perforation should result during the plunge step, this initial hesitation also permits detection of the perforation while it is still minute in size and not extended.

3) Peripheral cutting is initiated by a combination of knife movement and forceps rotation of the eye, depending more on the rotational component, concentrating on maintaining the proper knife position (Figure 9-20), and constantly watching for any appearance of aqueous humor indicating a perforation has occurred.

4) The incision is terminated in clear cornea just short of the limbus (0.5 mm) to prevent hemorrhage from the peripheral corneal vascular arcades (Figure 9-21). Each subsequent incision is made in similar fashion.

The cutting action in radial keratotomy consists of a combined movement of the knife as well as an opposite direction movement of the fixation forceps. The amount of knife vs. fixation forceps movement varies according to technique. It appears easier to perform a straight perpendicular incision by concentrating on maintaining a proper perpendicular position of the knife and relying on eye rotation by the fixation forceps for creating the incisions. Since intraocular pressure decreases with each incision, which can result in shallow incisions, compensatory pressure on the fixation forceps can be effectively applied, especially during the "plunge" phase of cutting.

Variations: The First Incision. The choice of the corneal meridian for the initial incision is controversial. Since the temporal cornea, especially the inferotemporal quadrant, is usually the thinnest, many surgeons incise this meridian last and the thicker nasal cornea first in an attempt to avoid having to abort surgery due to a significant perforation early in the case. Other surgeons incise the thinner temporal meridians first, reasoning that there may be an even greater risk of perforation by incising the thinner meridians last since the cornea becomes thinner throughout the course of surgery due to dehydration. In addition, by incising the thinnest meridians first, the thicker corneal areas should become thinner with time, resulting in a more uniform final incision depth all around. This debate is further complicated by the progressive decrease in intraocular pressure that occurs with each incision resulting in shallower incisions unless compensatory external pressure is applied to the eye. A third group of surgeons prefer to initiate surgery by incising the four cardinal meridians starting with either the vertical or horizontal meridians and finishing with four radials spaced symmetrically between the first four cardinal incisions.

Variations: Cutting from Periphery to Center. Fyodorov's original technique of radial keratotomy consisted of making the radial incisions from the periphery centrally. Using razor blade fragments from Sputnik blades which produced smooth, even cutting action, Fyodorov achieved a high degree of surgical control with this technique and his instrumentation. The primary advantage of cutting from the periphery centrally is the improved ability to produce the desired deep perpendicular incision-profile (Figure 9-22) at the edge of the optical zone, which is the area responsible for the majority of the observed surgical effect.[6,7] The primary disadvantage is the danger of inadvertently carrying an incision centrally beyond the optical zone border. In the United States, most radial keratotomies are performed cutting from the center peripherally because of this fear of cutting into the optical zone which may result in increased glare, decreased best corrected visual acuity, and possible resultant litigation. Nevertheless, there are American surgeons who utilize both metal and diamond knives and perform the surgery in the classic periphery to center cutting manner.

Variations: Fixation Devices. In addition to the two-point fixation forceps, single-point toothed forceps as well as the Kremer two-point fixation forceps (Figure 9-23) have been used. The Kremer forceps provide excellent immobilization and tortional control over the eye. In addition, less topical anesthetic is required for comfort since the eye is grasped at two points (six and 12 o'clock) simultaneously only once and the forceps is locked for the duration of the procedure. There is the ability to increase intraocular pressure by pressure on the forceps. Rotational ability is not as great as with conventional two-point fixation forceps.

Certain fixation rings, such as the Barraquer suction ring, usually require

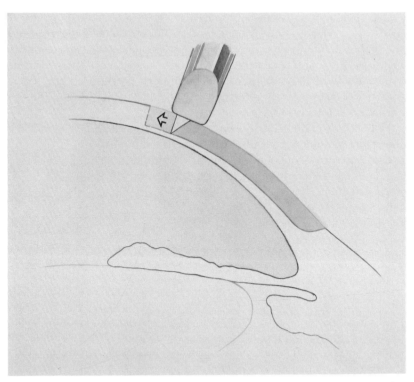

Figure 9-22. Diagram of perpendicular incision-profile at the optical zone obtained when cutting from the periphery centrally.

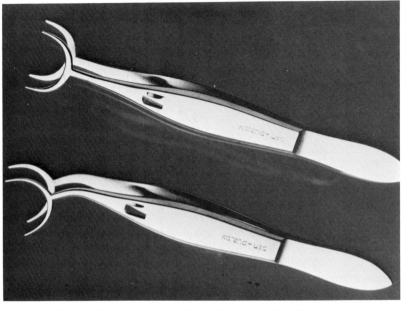

Figure 9-23. Kremer fixation forceps, straight and angled (preferred).

the use of a retrobulbar anesthetic for patient comfort. They do, however, provide both positional control as well as an improved ability to maintain adequate intraocular pressure throughout the surgical procedure to improve the ability to make the final incisions as deep as the first. With the Thornton ring, pressure is increased by downward pressure against the globe by the ring. The Barraquer suction ring elevates intraocular pressure to 60 mm Hg and maintains this pressure throughout the surgical procedure. Recently, Gelender[8] described a vacuum fixation ring that provides fixation of the globe and controls intraocular pressure "with only topical anesthesia." The stated disadvantages of most suction rings include the possibility of intraoperative loss of suction, vascular occlusion, increased intraoperative and postoperative chemosis, discomfort, subconjunctival hemorrhages, and increased initial rate of microperforations.

Sequence of Incisions. The classic sequence of incisions was governed by the belief that the cuts should be made 180° away from each other (Figure 9-24). However, if the surgery should have to be interrupted for any reason, it would be reasonable that the sequence of incisions should have a symmetrical effect on corneal topography. Therefore, it would appear that the sequence of incisions should be 90° away from each other (Figure 9-25).

In 16-incision cases, the second set of eight incisions is usually placed symmetrically between the initial eight radial cuts. The sequence employed for the second eight radials varies from the classic 180° approach to a simple sequential pattern. Some surgeons use a serial quadrant by quadrant technique from start to finish without making an initial set of eight symmetrical incisions. In all 16-incision cases, maintenance of adequate intraocular pressure by external pressure from the fixation forceps is important to prevent shallow incision depth in the later radial cuts (Figure 9-26).

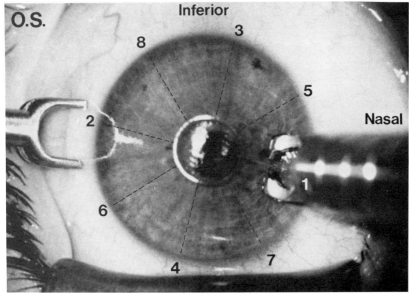

Figure 9-24. Photograph illustrating classic sequence of radial keratotomy incisions. Note last incision is in the inferotemporal quadrant (usually the thinnest).

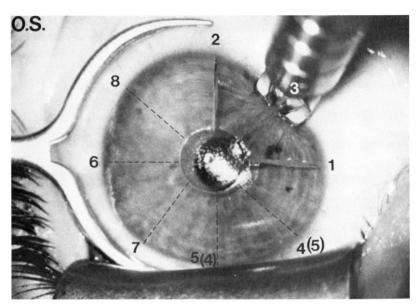

Figure 9-25A. Photograph of alternative sequence of incisions. Note that if an incision marker was not used, it is easier to maintain symmetry by reversing the order of incisions 4 and 5.

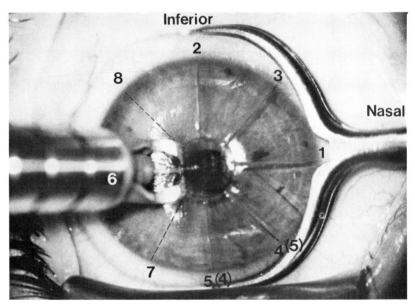

Figure 9-25B. In this left eye case when using the Kremer fixation forceps, incisions 1 through 5 are performed with the knife held in the right hand and fixation forceps in the left. The knife is then held in the left hand and forceps in the right for the final three incisions.

Verifying Incision Depth. Accurate intraoperative evaluation of the absolute depth of the incisions with a depth gauge is difficult. Corneal stroma swells with each incision resulting in the incisions appearing deeper than they really are. However, a hockey stick depth gauge instrument (Figure 9-27) can be used to identify the relatively shallow incisions. With

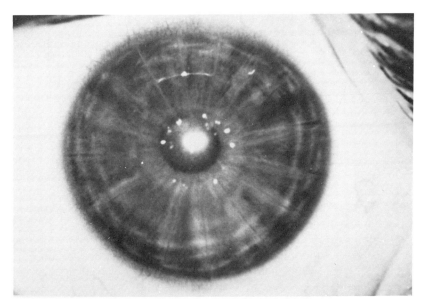

Figure 9-26. Intraoperative appearance of 16 incision case. External pressure applied with fixation forceps to maintain adequate intraocular pressure is important to insure proper depth of last eight incisions.

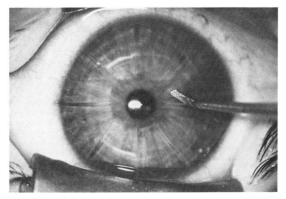

Figure 9-27A.

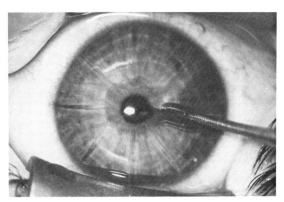

Figure 9-27B.

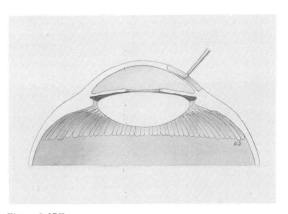

Figure 9-27C.

Figure 9-27A. Hockey stick depth gauge blade just above corneal incision.

Figure 9-27B. Depth gauge blade placed within corneal incision.

Figure 9-27C. Artist's illustration.

experience, intraoperative measurement of the depth of the incisions is neither necessary nor advisable because of the additional corneal trauma manipulating the incisions and possibility of epithelial seeding of the incisions.

Irrigation of the Incisions and Conclusion of Surgery. After completion of the desired number of incisions, the diamond blade is irrigated with distilled water to remove salts and organic debris and is carefully cleaned with a moist microsponge. Each incision is then gently tangentially irrigated with balanced salt solution through a 27 gauge cannula to remove epithelial cells, blood, and particulate debris (Figure 9-28). A broad spectrum antibiotic solution (e.g. tobramycin) is instilled together with a short acting cycloplegic such as cyclopentolate 1%. A steri-strip tape is used to close the eyelids followed by an eyepatch. Some surgeons leave the eye open (unless epithelial divots occurred) with instructions to instill antibiotic drops every few hours. Acetaminophen with codeine or equivalent oral analgesic is prescribed and the patient is instructed to return in 24 hours. The typical appearance of an eight-incision case is shown at one day, four weeks, and four years after surgery in Figure 9-29.

Deepening of Primary Incisions: The Second and Third Zones.
It is possible to obtain a greater effect from radial keratotomy surgery by deepening the periphery of the incisions since the corneal thickness increases toward the periphery. Fyodorov first described the technique (Figure 9-30). The amount of increased effect is variable and dependent on individual surgical technique. Schachar feels that the additional effect from peripheral redeepening is minimal.[9]

Technique. Having completed the primary incisions, the blade of the micrometer knife is extended or a second preset knife is obtained. The second zone mark placed previously is identified and each incision is deepened starting at this mark, recutting peripherally (Figure 9-31). A light touch is required together with eye rotation rather than excessive movement of the knife to prevent perforations and to keep the blade within the original incision. If a tertiary zone is cut, this is deepened by cutting from

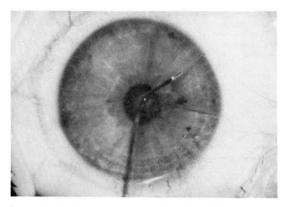

Figure 9-28A. Irrigation of corneal incision. Note irrigating cannula is held tangential to Descemet's membrane.

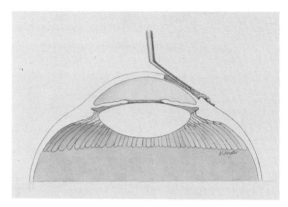

Figure 9-28B. Artist's illustration.

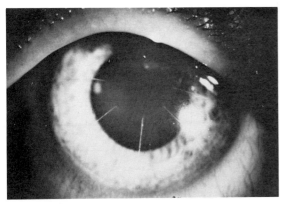

Figure 9-29A.

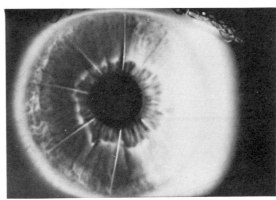

Figure 9-29B.

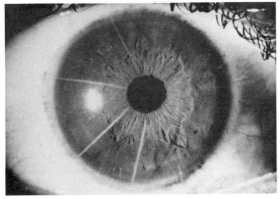

Figure 9-29A. Appearance of eight-incision case first day after surgery. Note fine punctate keratopathy from optical zone marker indentation.

Figure 9-29B. Scleral scatter photograph of same patient four weeks after surgery.

Figure 9-29C. Eight-incision case four years after surgery.

Figure 9-29C.

the periphery to the third zone mark (Figure 9-32). Some surgeons recut the entire length of the primary incision with the same micrometer blade setting in order to obtain greater depth and more effect from the surgery.[10]

Peripheral redeepening of the primary incisions is controversial. Those surgeons utilizing this technique support its effectiveness in obtaining an additional effect from the surgery. Those surgeons not using peripheral redeepening either contend it has no increased effect in their hands or feel that the disadvantages of this technique outweigh the advantage of the additional correction they are able to obtain. Disadvantages include increased risk of perforation, difficulty of staying in the same groove within the depth of the incision, and additional surgical trauma resulting in possible greater loss of corneal endothelial cells and increased glare/flare from excessive scarring.

Two-Stage Procedures. Radial keratotomy surgery can be planned as a two-stage procedure in certain specific cases. Some surgeons feel they can achieve a greater correction in 16-incision cases by performing eight incisions during the first stage of the procedure and subsequently adding

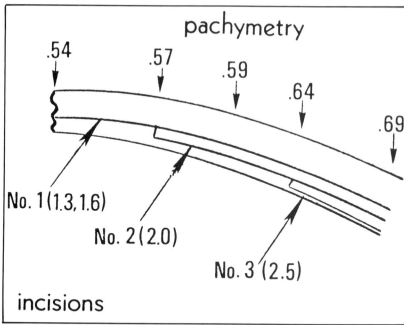

Figure 9-30A. Diagram of corneal cross section (pachymetry measurements between .54 mm centrally to .69 mm in the far periphery) illustrating Fyodorov's classic graded-incision surgical approaches. Surgical approach 1 involves single depth incisions. Approach 2 involves second zone peripheral deepening and approach 3 involves third zone free-hand deepening to Descemet's membrane.

1.3   one incision, P.C. - 0.08 (∽80%)*

1.6   ''   , P.C - 0.05 (∽90%)*

2.0   above, plus M.P. -   ''

2.5   above, plus 4 - 8 cuts to Descemet's

*adjust for blade type

Figure 9-30B. Fyodorov's four surgical factors (1.3, 1.6, 2.0, and 2.5) defining a particular surgical approach. Factor 1.3: Single incision with blade set at paracentral optical pachymetry minus 0.08 which is approximately equated to 80% observed corneal depth. Factor 1.6: Single incision with blade set at paracentral optical pachymetry minus 0.05 which is approximately 90% observed corneal depth. Factor 2.0: Single initial incisions as in Factor 1.6 with additional peripheral deepening of all incisions at blade setting of mid-peripheral optical pachymetry minus 0.05. Factor 2.5: Initial incisions and peripheral deepening as in Factor 2.0 with additional free-hand deepening to Descemet's membrane in four to eight incisions depending on degree of myopia.

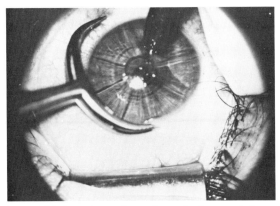

Figure 9-31. Second zone deepening at the 5 mm optical zone mark.

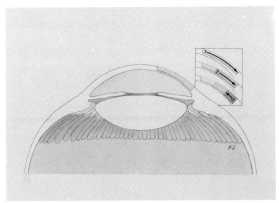

Figure 9-32. Diagram of three-step incision showing increasing depth of cut and direction primary, secondary, and tertiary incisions.

eight additional cuts at a later date, rather than performing 16 cuts during the initial surgery.[11] Another group of patients that may be suitable for staged surgery are those who experienced a significant unexplained overcorrection in their first eye, and the surgeon is attempting to produce binocularity with minimal overcorrection in the fellow eye. A third group that might benefit from staged surgery are certain patients with high risk factors (e.g. presbyopic male with high IOP) where overcorrection is of great concern. Staging the surgery has the advantage of somewhat more control over the final effect of surgery. Mathematical model analysis predicts that the first four incisions in an eight-incision case contribute approximately 60% of the effect while the first eight incisions of a 16-incision case are responsible for approximately 90% of the observed effect.[12] These percentage figures can be used to plan a two-stage procedure. Clinically, however, it appears that the predicted increase in the effect of the additional second set of incisions can be greater than anticipated if the initial incisions were shallow and a longer time interval of several months is allowed to pass between sets of incisions. Disadvantages of two-stage surgery include prolonged rehabilitation time, increased hospital or surgical facility costs to the patient, some degree of increased surgical trauma, and increased exposure to possible complications. Technical difficulties with secondary surgery are due to the difficulty in visualization of the primary incisions (especially in light colored irides where preoperative dilation is helpful) resulting in increased difficulty in exact placement of the optical zone marker over the previous optical zone and placement of the additional incisions symmetrically between the primary cuts. In cases where only four incisions were made, there may be a greater risk of inducing regular astigmatism.

Complications: Subconjunctival Hemorrhage, Corneal Vascular Arcade Hemorrhage, Epithelial Divots, Oblique Incisions, Sigmoid Incisions, Shallow Incisions, and Perforating Incisions. If a subconjunctival hemorrhage should occur before commencing the first corneal incision, direct pressure can be applied to the bleeding limbal vessel to stop the bleeding. If, however, a hemorrhage should occur after the incisions have been started, they should be completed before dealing with the bleeding vessel. By delaying, corneal thickness may change enough to result in varying depth incisions. Nicking of the pericorneal vascular arcades (Figure 9-33) is a frequent event and of no serious consequence providing the hemorrhage is stopped with direct pressure and the incision irrigated free of blood and debris with balanced salt solution before terminating the surgery.

Corneal epithelial defects occur much less frequently today with the use of diamond knives with highly polished blade guards than in the past with the use of blade breakers and razor blade fragments. Likewise, avoiding the use of cocaine drops which can loosen the epithelial cells will decrease the occurrence of these defects. Nevertheless, epithelial divots can occur and are best managed by careful unfolding and repositioning of the epithelial sheet over the defect at the conclusion of surgery. Usually there are no adverse sequelae, although the development of anterior membrane dystrophic changes in the area of the epithelial defect (Figure 9-34) and symptoms of recurrent epithelial erosions are possible.[13]

Oblique incisions result from less than perpendicular position of the

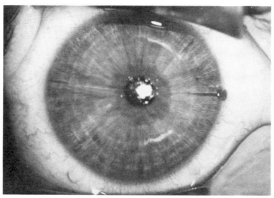

Figure 9-33A.

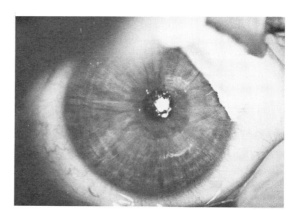

Figure 9-33B.

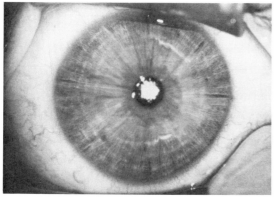

Figure 9-33C.

Figure 9-33A. Hemorrhage from nicked nasal incision.

Figure 9-33B. Pressure applied to bleeding vessel.

Figure 9-33C. Hemorrhage stopped.

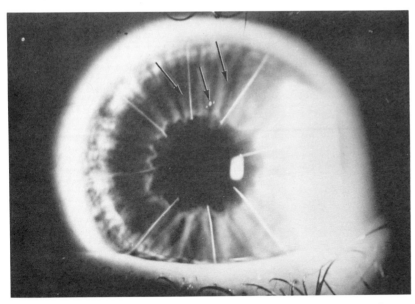

Figure 9-34. Corneal photograph of 37-year-old female following radial keratotomy. Surgery uneventful except for stripping of large sector of corneal epithelium when making 12 o'clock radial incision. Epithelium was replaced at the conclusion of surgery. Healing characterized by map-dot and fingerprint anterior membrane dystrophic changes of superior cornea (arrows). Map-dot changes eventually cleared. Fingerprint lines still present two and one-half years after surgery. Presently patient is asymptomatic and has uncorrected vision of 20/30, correctable to 20/20 with −0.25 + 1.00 × 180. Fellow eye underwent uneventful surgery one year later and has 20/20 uncorrected vision.

knife (Figure 9-35). Oblique incisions may be responsible for increased glare/flare especially if they are located close to the visual axis. They may also be too shallow, depending on the amount of shelving.

Concentrating on maintaining the knife blade normal to the corneal surface will avoid oblique cuts. Rotating the eye with the fixation forceps rather than moving the knife is also helpful. Sigmoid incisions are the result of torsional eye movements or non-linear knife movements. Torsional eye movements can be minimized by using two-point fixation forceps or fixation rings. Fortunately, although esthetically less than satisfying to the surgeon when viewed through the slit lamp, sigmoid incisions are compatible with a good visual result, providing the depth of the cut is adequate.

No universal agreement yet exists with respect to the precise optimal depth of radial keratotomy incisions. The incisions must be deep enough but the exact depth that will give a permanent predictable result is not known. Attempted incision depth placement varies between 85% to 95%[14,15] of the corneal thickness depending on the surgeon. All agree that shallow incisions produce less than the expected result and significantly more regression. Shallow incisions are almost inevitable at some point during the learning curve of radial keratotomy surgery. Shallow incisions can be the result of the surgeon's timidity in choosing a particular blade setting or failure to apply adequate pressure during the incision making

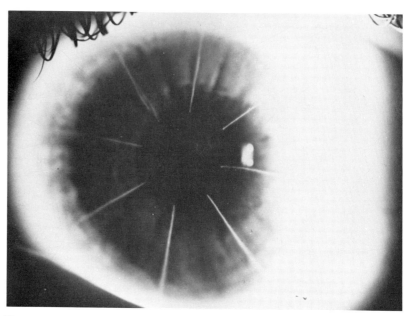

Figure 9-35. Oblique incision at 10:30 meridian.

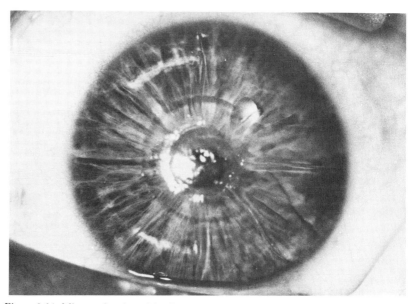

Figure 9-36. Microperforation with minute bead of aqueous humor occurring during peripheral deepening. Note second zone corneal indentation mark.

process. In other cases, the pachymetry measurements may have been inaccurate, the blade extension may not have been properly set, or the knife blade itself may have been dull. Sixteen-incision cases require compensatory pressure from the fixation forceps or fixation ring to produce sufficient firmness in the globe toward the end of the case to insure deep incisions. If a corneal perforation occurs, intraocular pressure may be decreased sufficiently to make it impossible to make subsequent incisions of adequate depth. The depth measurement gauge can be used to approximate the relative depths of the incisions. Shallow incisions can then be recut. However, recutting can produce excessive scarring. Here again, the best treatment is prevention: obtain a reliable, accurate pachymeter and

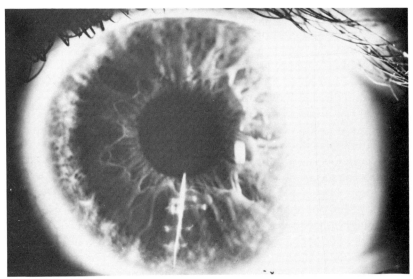

Figure 9-37A. Scleral scatter photograph of macroperforation in 33 year old female (initial refraction: −6.75 + 1.75 × 85) two months after removal of 10-0 nylon sutures (refraction: −3.75 + 1.25 × 75).

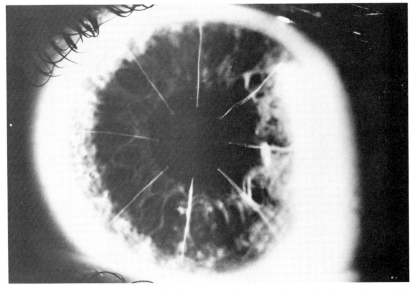

Figure 9-37B. Patient in Figure 9-37A after seven additional incisions added (optical zone 3.00 mm) three months after initial surgery. Visual acuity six months after additional cuts added: 20/30 without correction, 20/20 with −1.00 + 1.25 × 80.

calibrated knife that is properly set and plunge deeply and with faith in your instruments.

Perforations can be divided into microperforations or macroperforations. Microperforations usually permit continuation of the surgery without significant loss of aqueous and intraocular pressure. If a microperforation is noted by the sudden appearance of fluid within the incision (Figure 9-36), the surgery is momentarily stopped and both the incision and knife tip are dried with a microsponge. The microperforation will usually self seal. If the eye is firm enough, the other incisions away from the perforation are completed, leaving the incomplete incision for last. Usually, the same knife setting is used after verifying the correct extension of the blade on the measuring gauge since the loss of aqueous humor into the incision usually causes some degree of local corneal swelling. If the incision is continued immediately in spite of evidence of a microperforation, there is danger of extending the internal opening to macroproportions. At the conclusion of the surgery, incisions with a perforation should be carefully irrigated, if at all, to prevent the possibility of inadvertent introduction of material into the anterior chamber.

If a macroperforation should occur, surgery usually cannot be continued because of the marked loss of aqueous humor and intraocular pressure. Interrupted 10-0 nylon sutures are used to effect a tight closure, burying the knots within the cornea. If necessary, the anterior chamber should be deepened with balanced salt solution to be certain the incision is free of any iris tissue. Sutures are removed as early as possible to minimize scarring yet insure adequate healing (usually two to four weeks). The surgery can be completed three months after the initial macroperforation (Figure 9-37).

In all cases of suspected or obvious perforations, subconjunctival injection of tobramycin 20 mg is given in the following fashion. After the surgery is completed, additional tetracaine drops are placed in the inferotemporal conjunctival cul-de-sac. One-half cc of lidocaine 1% is slowly injected through a 27-gauge needle anesthetizing the inferotemporal quadrant. Tobramycin is then injected into this anesthetized area through the same needle.

References

1. Fyodorov SN, Durnev VV: Operation of Dosaged Dissection of Corneal Circular Ligament in Cases of Myopia of Mild Degree. *Ann Ophthalmol* 11:1885-1889, 1979.
2. Hoffer K: Interview on "Medical Portfolio for Ophthalmologists", 1983.
3. Elander R: Radial Keratotomy Manual, Jules Stein Institute.
4. Saltz J, Azen S, Berstein J, Caroline P, Villaseñor R, Schanzlin D: Evaluation and Comparison of Sources of Variability in the Measurement of Corneal Thickness with Ultrasonic and Optical Pachymeters. *Ophthal Surg* 14:750-754, 1983.
5. Kremer FB: Pre- and Postoperative Topographical Corneal Pachymetry. *In:* Radial Keratoplasty, Schachar RA, Levy NS, Schachar L, (eds), Denison, TX: LAL Publishing, 1983, p 207.
6. Schachar RA, Black TD, Huang T: *Understanding Radial Keratotomy*, Denison, TX: LAL Publishing, 1981, p 25.
7. Deitz MR: Radial Keratotomy—Which Variables Affect the Outcome the Most. *In:* Refractive Keratoplasty, Schachar RA, Levy NS, Schachar L, (eds), Denison, TX: LAL Publishing, 1983, p 266.
8. Gelender H: Vacuum Fixation Ring for Radial Keratotomy. *Ophthal Surg* 15:126-127, 1984.
9. Schachar RA, et al: op cit, pp 25-27.

10. Sanders D, (ed): *Radial Keratotomy*, Thorofare, NJ: Slack, Inc, 1984, p 43.
11. Schachar RA, et al: op cit, p 62.
12. Ibid, p 21.
13. Rowsey JJ, Balyeat HD: Radial Keratotomy: Preliminary Report of Complications. *Ophthal Surg* 13:29, 1982.
14. Schachar RA, et al: op cit, p 138.
15. Sanders D: op cit, pp 39-51.

Chapter 10

Control of Astigmatism Using Corneal Incisions

Robert E. Fenzl MD, FACS

CONTROL OF ASTIGMATISM
USING CORNEAL INCISIONS

Duke-Elder defines astigmatism as that type of refractive anomaly in which no point focus is formed. This anomaly is due to the unequal refraction of incident light in different meridians by the dioptric system of the eye. While Duke-Elder's definition is probably one of the most concise, an expanded definition is necessary for greater understanding. Although irregular astigmatism is a consideration, we are more concerned in refractive surgery with regular astigmatism. Regular astigmatism is best considered as being produced by a toroidal surface rather than a spherical refractive surface of the eye (Figure 10-1). No single focal point of light is obtained on a toroidal surface and, therefore, the image is blurred.

The basic concept of astigmatism is a simple one (the cornea is shaped like a football and is therefore nonspherical). However, the myriad of terms used in the description of astigmatism have made it a confusing topic. From a practical standpoint, astigmatism described as "with-the-rule" is the most common type (Figure 10-2). "With-the-rule" astigmatism is pres-

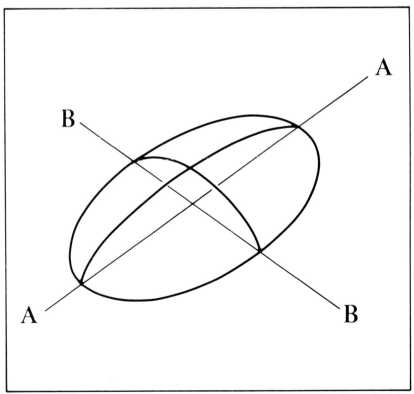

Figure 10-1. Toroidal surface as would be seen in a cornea with astigmatism. The axis of the steepest meridian runs through B and the axis of the flatter meridian is through A.

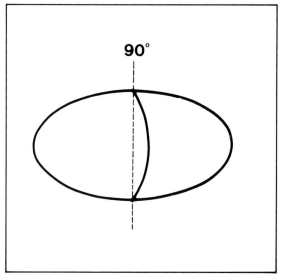

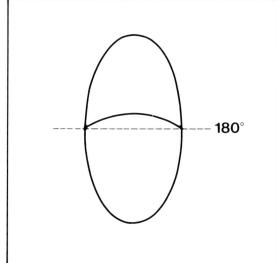

Figure 10-2. Shape of a cornea with "with-the-rule" astigmatism. The axis of the steepest meridian is at 90°.

Figure 10-3. Shape of a cornea with "against-the-rule" astigmatism. The axes of the steepest meridian is at 180°.

ent when the steepest meridian is at the 90° axis, or the "football" is lying on its side. In this instance, when dealing with refractions in plus cylinder, the plus axis is closest to the 90° meridian. The exact opposite is true with "against-the-rule" astigmatism; this is the less common presentation and is similar to a football standing on end. In this instance, the axis of the plus cylinder is closest to 180°, the steepest meridian (Figure 10-3).

History

The historical record of astigmatism began in the early 1800's. The English scientist, Thomas Young, was the first to recognize astigmatism as a defect in his own vision in 1801. It was not until 1827 that the astronomer Sir George Biddell Airy, while studying his own problem of astigmatism, was able to have an optician named Fuller grind a lens correcting his astigmatism. In 1864 Donders wrote the earliest landmark paper on optics in relationship to astigmatism. Attempts to surgically correct astigmatism, especially that found after cataract surgery, came relatively soon after Donder's classic paper. The earliest known attempts were made by Snellen[1] in 1869. Snellen described anterior corneal incisions to reduce the high postoperative astigmatism found in cataract surgery done without sutures. Others who attempted to flatten the steepest corneal meridian, as Snellen did included Bates[2] in 1894, who used an unsutured corneal wedge resection, and Sato[3] in 1939, who attempted radial corneal incisions. The first attempt to steepen the flattest corneal meridian was described by Lans[4] in 1898, using corneal cautery. This attempt was followed by sutured wedge resections of the cornea by Poyales[5] in 1953, and of the sclera by Barraquer[6] in 1956. All of these procedures were eventually abandoned because of the poor reliability and unpredictability. The first significant modern attempts in the control of postoperative astigmatism began with the work of Richard Troutman.[7,8] His description of the changes that occurred during cataract wound formation and subsequent suturing was a quantum step in the understanding of postcataract astigmatism. Additionally, Troutman's description of corneal wedge resections and relaxing incisions, which Krachmer and I[9] recently evaluated, have been the foundation of correcting postoperative corneal transplant astigmatism (Figures 10-4 and 10-5). (See Chapter 11 for a more complete description of wedge resections and relaxing incisions.)

A greater understanding of the nature, prevention, and control of corneal astigmatism came with the introduction of the surgical keratometer. While the first units were of a qualitative nature, the introduction of the Terry quantitative unit was a significant advancement. This instrument allowed real time understanding of the effects of suturing and incisions on the cornea along with a true measurement of this curvature change. Studies by Terry, Kratz, Blaydes, and others have shown the usefulness of the keratometer in controlling and adjusting postoperative corneal astigmatism.

Despite all the previous groundwork, it took the development of radial keratotomy by Fyodorov[10] to show that incisional corneal surgery could change the central corneal curvature in a predictable manner not only for the correction of myopia but also for the correction of astigmatism. Since Fyodorov's first cases in Russia in 1973 and the first cases in the United States by Bores in 1979, the knowledge and understanding of the ability of incisional surgery to alter the shape of the cornea has multiplied in an almost exponential fashion.

Myopia and Astigmatism

The introduction of radial keratotomy in the late 1970's started a new era in refractive surgery. Not only were the interests of individual surgeons stimulated in the area of refractive surgery for myopia, but the specific procedures described by Fyodorov for astigmatism correction, with and without myopia, rejuvenated general interest in this field. Though all the procedures described by Fyodorov have either been replaced or modified, the principles that longer and more numerous radial incisions differentially flatten the meridian and the addition or tangential incisions alone or, more importantly, in combination with radial incisions, can again differentially flatten that corneal meridian were essential for the development of modern day astigmatism correction.

It is important to understand both the local and peripheral effects of incisions in the cornea, both sutured and unsutured. It is with great difficulty that most residents learn the principle that a tight suture causes steepening of the central cornea. These refractive and keratometric readings postoperatively don't seem to correlate with the apparent corneal curvature change at the time the suture is being tied. This is because of the differential between local and more distant effects of suture tightening on the cornea. In doing so, there is a shortening of the cord length of the cornea in that meridian and, therefore, a central steepening of the cornea.

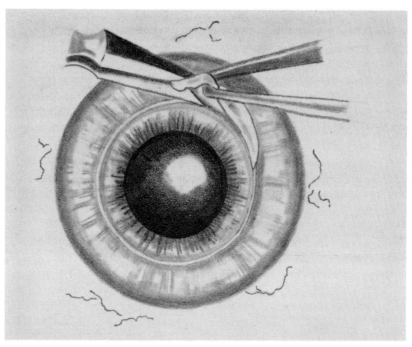

Figure 10-4. Wedge resection at host-graft interface to correct post-keratoplasty astigmatism.

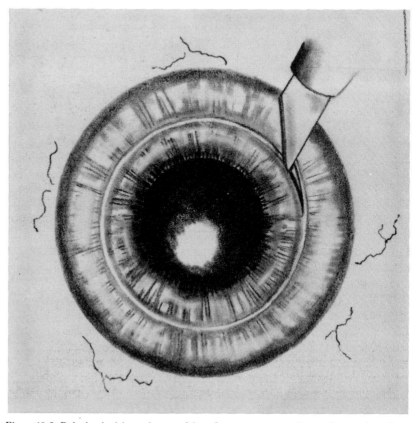

Figure 10-5. Relaxing incision at host-graft interface to correct post-keratoplasty astigmatism.

The principle of a loose suture corresponds more closely with the effect of both radial and transverse incisions on the peripheral cornea used in astigmatism correction. In all of these cases there is a loosening or weakening of the peripheral corneal structure, and the intraocular pressure causes the surrounding tissue to expand and steepen. In doing so, the cord length is lengthened in that meridian or, in myopic surgery, in the entire peripheral cornea, and the central corneal curvature is flattened. This is best represented in a spherical myopia case by the "donut" analogy (Figure 10-6). This differential between the local and more distant effects of corneal incisions is extremely important. When considering the principles of astigmatism correction, increased flattening is necessary in the axis of the positive cylinder or 90° from the axis of the minus cylinder.

During the past five years, I have attempted many modifications of radial keratotomy to more effectively allow correction of significant degrees of myopic astigmatism. In astigmatism combined with myopia of degrees between 1 diopter and 3 diopters, I have found a modification of Fyodorov's original TR procedure is most useful (Figure 10-7). The amount of surgery to be performed is calculated by attempting to correct the refractive sphere, not spherical equivalent, with the patient's refraction expressed in *minus* cylinder form, using a standard radial keratotomy procedure. In the majority of cases this would mean an eight-incision procedure but it can vary between six and 12 incisions. This is the same principle we use in hard contact lens fitting where astigmatism can be ignored due to the tear film generated under the contact lens. The degree of refractive cylinder or astigmatism is corrected by placing two transverse incisions on either side of the optical zone on the axis of the steepest meridian.

The incisions sit at an optical zone of approximately 7 mm to 7.5 mm. Determination of their length is done on a percentage of the distance from one eight-incision radial to the next. This allows for variation in corneal diameter and also allows for variation in optical zone if a smaller or larger optical zone is desired to attempt more or less correction. It is important to start an incision as far away from a radial as is possible and to direct that incision towards the next radial, entering it on one side but not extending all the way through the radial incision. Entering that radial incision, in my hands, gives more correction than if the radial was not entered. It is not advisable to totally cross the radial incision and exit to the other side since this causes a "fishmouth" type wound, which in a number of cases has led to difficulty in wound healing.

This procedure was originally developed empirically with the data being evaluated retrospectively. After reviewing approximately 100 cases with a number of variations on the same theme, the present procedure was selected as having the best fit. A minimum starting astigmatism of 1 diopter and a maximum of 3.25 D were evaluated prospectively in 50 cases with a follow up of at least one year. With the distance between one radial incision and another at the optical zone of 7.5 mm being defined as X, it was determined that one-half X accounted for between 1 diopter and 1.5 diopters of astigmatism correction. If the transverse incision on each side was extended from just before entering one radial incision to the entrance of the other radial incision, in other words X, approximately 2.5 diopters to 3 diopters of astigmatism correction could be obtained. In the 50 cases so

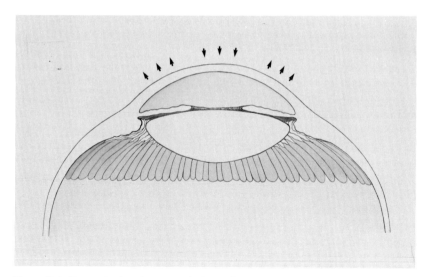

Figure 10-6. Forces shaping the cornea during radial keratotomy. Peripheral steepening with central flattening simulates the shape of a donut.

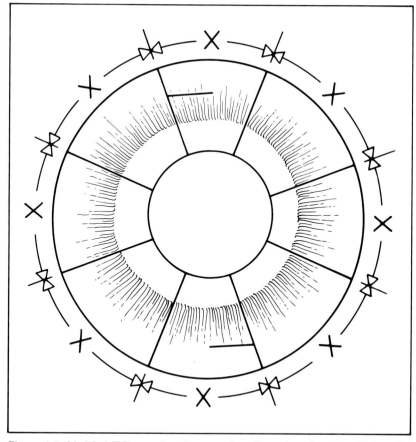

Figure 10-7. Modified T-R procedure for correction of myopic astigmatism. Eight radial incisions are used as well as T- (transverse-) incisions. The T-incisions in this case transverse approximately one-half of the distance, X, between radial incisions. This should correct between 1 diopter and 1.5 diopters of astigmatism.

evaluated on a prospective basis, average astigmatism was 1.95 diopters preoperatively, and postoperatively the average astigmatism was .47 diopters. These results were not evaluated by vector analysis since from both patient's and surgeon's point of view it was of little importance whether the patient went from a diopter and a half of astigmatism in one meridian to a half a diopter of astigmatism in a meridian 90° away or if the patient went from one and a half diopters of astigmatism in one meridian to a half a diopter of astigmatism in that meridian. The ultimate result of a residual of one half a diopter of astigmatism was the important consideration. As in radial keratotomy, there was some variation, but the most important was noted in cases where the incisions were not of adequate depth, i.e., less than 90%. It is extremely important at the time of surgery to measure the corneal thickness with ultrasonic pachymetry directly over the area to be cut. Peripheral corneal thickness varies to even a greater degree than central and paracentral corneal thickness, and increasing the thickness of the blade a standard amount over that used for the radial incisions did not give consistent depths. It is also extremely important to make sure the footplate of the blade is perfectly parallel with the peripheral corneal curvature. A number of earlier cases, because of natural tendency, were placed more parallel to the central corneal curvature and, therefore, the incisions were long but angulated and were not adequately deep.

Low and Moderate Degrees of Corneal Astigmatism

The idea of using corneal incisions to flatten the cornea is not a new one.[1] The use of relaxing incisions in the keratoplasty wound for high posttransplant astigmatism has been well defined by Troutman,[7] Krachmer[9] and others. These same transverse relaxing incisions were described in the earliest papers by Fyodorov.[10] As a corneal Fellow, I had the opportunity to evaluate relaxing incisions and wedge resections as they relate to postkeratoplasty astigmatism. In early private practice, prior to the published works of Fyodorov, I worked on the possibility of using relaxing incisions to reduce postcataract astigmatism. A relatively fixed protocol was set dealing with patients having a minimum of 2.5 diopters and a maximum of 6 diopters of postcataract astigmatism. All patients were handled in a similar manner using four relaxing incisions, two on either side of the optical zone at the steepest meridian. The incisions extended 3 mm in length. The two most central incisions sat on an optical zone of 6 mm, the two more peripheral incisions were 0.5 mm from its companion and of identical length (Figure 10-8). As in other refractive surgical procedures, pachymetry readings were taken over the area to be incised and attempted depths of 90% or better were calculated.

Evaluation of this procedure with all patients at least one year postoperative showed an average astigmatism correction of slightly over 3.25 diopters. This ranged anywhere from as little as 0.5 diopters of change to as high as 6.25 diopters of change with 89% of the patients ranging from between 2 diopters and 4 diopters of astigmatism correction. The correction match was somewhat variable with the higher degrees of astigmatism sometimes obtaining the lower degrees of correction. For this reason, I have limited the use of the procedure to patients with less than 4.5 diopters of astigmatism and usually expect between 2 diopters and 4 diopters of change.

These results correspond closely with results obtained by Fyodorov and Fyodorov[14] using one relaxing incision on each side of the steep meridian with an optical zone averaging approximately 5 mm and incisions of 4 mm to 5 mm in length. The two Fyodorovs' reported results were a change of 3.26 diopters plus or minus 0.34 diopters in a similar patient group.

My experience with parallel incisions in the axis of the steepest meridians, which has been described by S.N. Fyodorov as the L Procedure, have not been so rewarding. The results have been inconsistent and variable with little ultimate correction. This is also confirmed by Fyodorov and Fyodorov.[14] In a similar patient population to the T-incisions, L-incisions only decreased corneal astigmatism by 1.15 diopters plus or minus 0.19 diopter.

Relaxing incisions, as classically described, can be of great assistance in reducing postkeratoplasty corneal astigmatism. T-incisions likewise can be used for high postoperative astigmatism after cataract surgery. Both procedures have the one problem of poor predictability but they seldom overcorrect and, therefore, are a simple and easy way to handle small degrees of postoperative astigmatism.

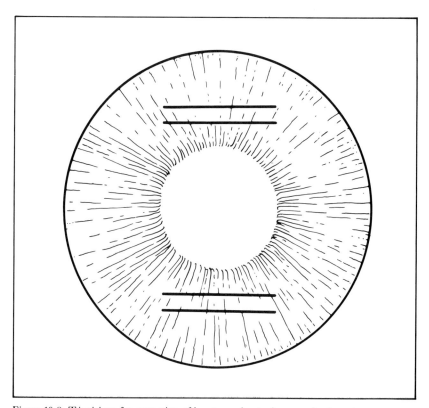

Figure 10-8. T-incisions for correction of low to moderate degrees of astigmatism.

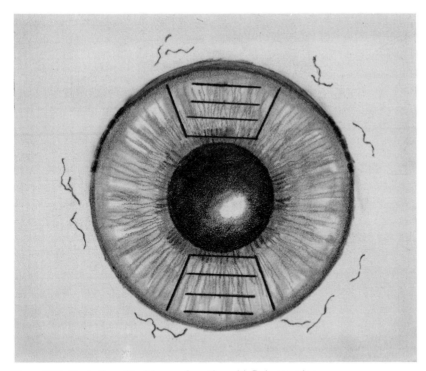

Figure 10-9. Illustration of incision configuration with Ruiz procedure.

Correction of High Astigmatism

The correction of pure astigmatism and the combination of myopia and high astigmatism, greater than 3 diopters, has been a much more difficult problem. The use of single and double relaxing incisions in pure astigmatism and the use of TR and RL procedures did not produce consistently reproducible results in these two categories. Many surgeons were attempting the combination of radial and transverse incisions to accomplish this goal, but the work of Luis Ruiz marked a milestone in this endeavor.

Ruiz combined short multiple tangential incisions on each side of the optical zone at the steepest meridian flanked by radial incisions. This approach produced a way of handling moderate to high corneal astigmatism both alone and in combination with the correction of myopia at the time of radial keratotomy surgery (Figure 10-9). Ruiz's original description was of five equally spaced tangential incisions of 2 mm to 2.5 mm in length on either side of the optical zone flanked on either side by a radial incision for a total of 14 incisions. He also presented tables of degrees of correction depending on the depth of incisions. This method has been modified for use in the United States by myself and a number of other surgeons by using four tangential incisions on either side along with the radials and carrying the depth of the incisions to 90% or better. As in radial keratotomy, the optical zones do not go smaller than 3 mm though Ruiz has described optical zones as small as 2.5 mm. Optical zones smaller than 3 mm cause

TABLE 10-1
RUIZ PROCEDURE MODIFIED TABLE

Optical Zone Size	Diopter Change
5.0 mm	2.0-3.0
4.5 mm	3.5-4.5
4.0 mm	5.0-6.0
3.5 mm	6.5-7.5
3.0 mm	8.0-9.0

All incisions 90% or greater. 30 year old patient base

significant optical aberrations from the incisions and unstable optical caps. Approximate correction obtained with varying size optical zones can be seen in the accompanying table (Table 10-1). This must be corrected for age and other factors as in radial keratotomy.

With the use of the Ruiz complex of incisions, corneal curvature changes from as small as 2 diopters to as great as 14 diopters of correction can be obtained in a relatively predictable fashion. In a series of 50 patients followed by me for at least one year, 85% were within 1.25 diopters of expected results.

This concept can be carried over to a patient with myopic astigmatism. In these cases the Ruiz procedure is placed first with its optical zone determined by using the astigmatism found in minus cylinders and placed on the steepest axis. The optical zone obtained for the radial incision is calculated using the sphere found in minus cylinder form. With the use of this combined procedure, myopia ranging from 2 diopters to 5.5 diopters and up to 8 D of concomitant astigmatism has been corrected (Figure 10-10).

Alignment of Astigmatism

All of the procedures that we have discussed in relation to the correction of astigmatism have used the principal of flattening the steepest corneal meridian. To accomplish this, it is essential that the incisions are placed directly on this meridian. In refraction it is taught that the power of a cylinder cannot be obtained until the proper axis is found. If astigmatism correction is attempted on an axis other than the correct one, a resultant astigmatism will be obtained. This is also true in the process of refractive corneal surgery. For this reason the use of an optical reticle is essential.

Accurate keratotomy readings and refraction are taken on the patient. The refraction must be extremely accurate since there are occasionally discrepancies between the axis of astigmatism keratometrically and of that refractively. This is most often due to secondary lenticular astigmatism.

When in doubt and after being sure of the measurements, the axis and degree of astigmatism should be taken from the patient's refraction. It is the refraction that the patient will ultimately see through and not his keratometric readings. Therefore the refraction should be the basis for correction. The patient is then thoroughly examined by biomicroscopy. The slit lamp which is used should possess an optical reticle. A prominent limbal blood vessel, iris crypt, or freckle is noted in the chart and its degree position is also noted. If for some reason there is no prominent feature that can be marked as far as its axis, then a small amount of methylene blue placed on the conjunctiva at the limbus superiorly at the 90° position will work. This is recorded in the chart and the planned surgical procedure is drawn accurately, placing the appropriate incisions in the indicated meridian. The drawing is then used in the operating room where an identical reticle is placed in the microscope ocular, the reticle is centered using the preplaced mark or positioning characteristic of the eye, and the appropriate angle can then be found and the procedure properly aligned.

If these precautions are not taken, it is very easy at the time of surgery for the astigmatism to be placed as much as 25° from the desired axis because of malpositioning of the microscope or torsion of the eye due to oblique muscle action. It is also important to draw the procedure out in a mapped fashion prior to entering the operating room, as is done in retinal detachment surgery. More than one surgeon has placed his astigmatism

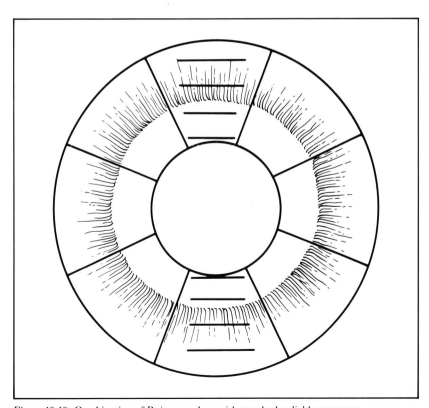

Figure 10-10. Combination of Ruiz procedure with standard radial keratotomy.

procedure 90° from the appropriate axis and actually increased the patient's astigmatism rather than decreasing it, because he failed to map out the procedure in advance.

Optical reticles of this type are available through Zeiss suppliers for Zeiss slit lamps or microscopes as a matched pair in 10× power, or an inexpensive individual reticle designed by me can be obtained for all major brands of slit lamps and microscopes through Dioptics of Irvine, California (Figure 10-11).

Complications

As in any surgical procedure of the eye, the ultimate complication is total loss of vision. To my knowledge the only marked loss of vision obtained in radial keratotomy and similar procedures has come from the retrobulbar injection of the optic nerve. Cataract formation and endophthalmitis have been reported,[11] and a number of cases of poorly placed optical zones have led to irregular astigmatism.[12]

Since the procedures for astigmatism are often performed on aphakic patients, corneal perforation can lead to the complication of vitreous to the wound which has been described by Binder.[13] In my own practice I have encountered only one significant complication. That complication occurred in the case of a Ruiz procedure where both the first and second

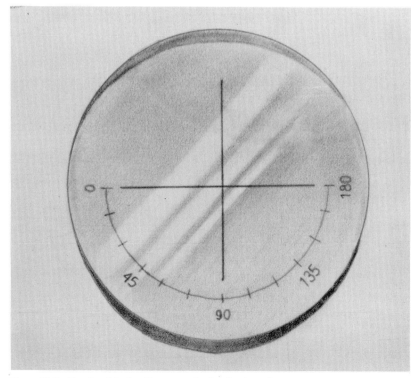

Figure 10-11. Fenzl reticle for alignment of axis of astigmatism.

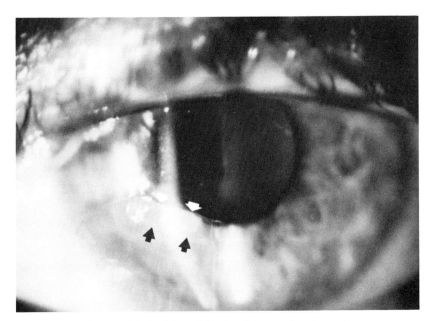

Figure 10-12. Edematous block of tissue following Ruiz procedure (arrows).

tangential incisions were connected with one of the radial incisions because of a movement of the patient's eye. The resultant rectangle of tissue became extremely edematous (Figure 10-12). Eventually, because of lack of epithelialization and edema, the tissue was excised in a lamellar fashion parallel with surrounding corneal surface. Although that area has developed a superficial haze, the surface has healed well and the patient has obtained an excellent optical result.

As in surgery for myopia alone, the major complication encountered in these procedures is poor correction. I have four postcataract patients who, despite what was calculated to be an adequate procedure for the amount of astigmatism, and good incisional depth, obtained little or no change in central corneal curvature. I also have two patients whose astigmatism was reduced in half although the total amount of change was 1½ times expected; the resultant astigmatism was 90° from their initial astigmatism; therefore, they obtained a significant overcorrection. These problems are not isolated to the Ruiz procedure since both undercorrections and overcorrections of similar amounts have been obtained by myself in the use of relaxing incisions following keratoplasty.

Conclusions

Although there has been some controversy over the use of surgery to correct myopia, it has never been questioned that moderate to high degrees of astigmatism—either postcataract, postcorneal transplant surgery, or naturally occurring astigmatism—are a significant optical handicap and that surgery is an appropriate means of correcting these defects. Until the last few years, there has been no accurate way of accomplishing this objective on a regular basis. The procedures that I have described for the correction of astigmatism alone or the correction of myopia and astigmatism at the same time have accomplished consistent optical corrections in all but a few patients. No loss of vision has occurred and no significant complications have been noted.

This is not to say that we have solved the problem of astigmatism. Although the procedures described are accurate, they are not perfect, and this is surely our goal. We can consistently flatten the cornea with the described procedures, but our ability to steepen the cornea has been less rewarding. Procedures such as wedge resections, microwedge resections, and sliding scleral flaps do accomplish this but in a very crude and unpredictable manner. With increased knowledge and technology as well as the use of new tools such as the Eximer Laser and corneal inserts, it is hoped that even greater predictability will be accomplished in our procedures for flattening the cornea and new and better procedures will be available for steepening the cornea.

References

1. Snellen H: Die Richtung der Hauptmeridiane des astigmatischen Auges. *Albrecht Von Graefes Arch Klin Exp Ophthalmol* 15:199-207, 1869.
2. Bates WH: A Suggestion of an Operation to Correct Astigmatism. *Arch Ophthalmol* 23:9-13, 1894.
3. Sato T: Posterior Incision of Cornea. *Am J Ophthalmol* 33:943-948, 1950.
4. Lans LJ: Experimentelle Untersuchungen uber die Entstehung von Astigmatismus durch nicht-perforirende Corneawunden. *Albrecht Von Graefes Arch Klin Exp Ophthalmol* 45:117-152, 1898.
5. Poyales I: Actas I Congreso Oftalmologico Latino, Rome, Arte della Stampa, 1953.
6. Barraquer J, Munos A: Lamellar Scleral Resection: Indications and technique. *Am J Ophthalmol* 41:92-98, 1956.
7. Troutman RC: Astigmatic Considerations in Corneal Graft. *Ophthalmic Surg* 10:21-26, 1979.
8. Troutman RC: *Microsurgery of the Anterior Segment of the Eye.* St. Louis: CV Mosby Co., 1977, p 286.
9. Krachmer JH, Fenzl RE: Surgical Correction of High Postkeratoplasty Astigmatism: Relaxing incisions vs. wedge resections. *Arch Ophthalmol* 98:1400-1402, 1980.
10. Fyodorov SM, Furney VV: Operation of Dosaged Dissection of Corneal Circular Ligament in Cases of Myopia of Mild Degree. *Ann Ophthalmol* 1979; 11:1885-1890.
11. Gelender H, Flynn HW, Jr, Mandelbaum SH: Bacterial Endophthalmitis Resulting from Radial Keratotomy. *Am J Ophthalmol* 93:323-326, 1982.
12. Rowsey JJ, Balyeat HD: Preliminary Results and Complications of Radial Keratotomy. *Am J Ophthalmol* 1982; 93:437-455.
13. Stainer GA, Binder PS: Vitreous Wick Syndrome Following a Corneal Relaxing Incision. *Ophthalmic Surgery* 12:567-570, 1981.
14. Fyodorov IS, Fyodorov SN: Surgical Correction of Corneal Astigmatism of Intraocular Lens Patients by the Method of Anterior Dosaged Keratotomy. Long term results. In press.

Chapter 11

Correction of Post-Keratoplasty Astigmatism

Richard L. Lindstrom, MD
G. William Lavery, MD

CORRECTION OF
POST-KERATOPLASTY ASTIGMATISM

The correction of refractive errors including astigmatism through the use of optical devices such as spectacles and contact lenses has always been a major part of every ophthalmologist's practice. A growing understanding of the etiology of corneal astigmatism has made it apparent that every surgical ophthalmologist is a refractive surgeon as well. Significant astigmatism may be induced following common surgical procedures including penetrating keratoplasty. In many cases the astigmatism may be minimized through appropriate incision and suturing techniques but, in some cases, excessive astigmatism develops. While the eye can often be visually rehabilitated through the use of spectacles or specialized contact lens, fitting some patients will require a surgical attempt to correct the high astigmatism.

In this chapter surgical techniques which have proven useful to the authors for the correction of high residual postoperative astigmatism following keratoplasty will be described. No attempt will be made to exhaustively review the history of refractive surgery for the correction of astigmatism, but appropriate references are provided for the interested reader. Primarily, the authors' personal experience and approach to postoperative astigmatism will be presented. The principles presented should be adapted to each surgeon's technique and experience.

Relaxing Incision

Introduction. The relaxing incision technique for the reduction of post-keratoplasty astigmatism is currently very popular. Most corneal surgeons have more experience with this approach than any other. Ophthalmic surgeons and several authors have reviewed their results utilizing this technique.[1-7] In the average patient a relaxing incision is capable of correcting four to five diopters of astigmatism with a range of zero to 10 diopters. This technique has the advantage of being relatively simple to perform, requiring only an office procedure and topical anesthesia. In addition, the postoperative recovery period is relatively short and the improvement in refractive status can be rapid and dramatic.

We have found the major disadvantages of this technique to be significant undercorrection and overcorrection. The operation is relatively unpredictable: an identical operation in one patient achieves a minimal effect with significant undercorrection while another patient achieves a large effect with significant overcorrection. Second, we have created several inadvertent perforations, some of which have required suturing. Finally, some patients develop a prolonged instability of the corneal topography with fluctuating keratometry as the graft appears to migrate during healing.

Nonetheless, this technique is still the most time tested and has proved useful in many surgeon's hands.

Operative Technique. The patient's refractive error is evaluated carefully preoperatively through the use of refraction, keratometry, and corneoscopy. We have found the relaxing incision technique to effectively flatten the steeper meridian and steepen the flatter meridian an equal amount. This means that the postoperative change in spherical equivalent is negligible. For example, if preoperatively a patient has a refractive error of $-3.00 +6.00 \times 90$ ($+3.00 -6.00 \times 180$) with keratometry readings of $40.00/46.00 \times 90$ and postoperatively the patient obtains a perfect result, the final spherical equivalent will be plano with keratometry readings of $43.00/43.00$ following surgery. This operation therefore will not correct any residual hyperopia or myopia.

The refraction, keratometry, and corneoscopy commonly performed each give the surgeon a different impression of the corneal topography. As refractions are often quite difficult and inaccurate in keratoplasty patients, we tend to rely primarily on keratometry and corneoscopy in planning our operation. The corneoscopy picture will often graphically demonstrate areas where cicatricial wound healing has resulted in significant corneal distortion. In some cases this poor wound healing will only be on one side of the graft host interface and a single relaxing incision will be satisfactory. In most cases relaxing incisions must be performed on both sides of the graft host interface in the axis of the steepest corneal meridian.

We prefer to perform the operation utilizing an operating microscope with a quantitative surgical keratometer. We feel this approach increases the accuracy of the procedure and may improve the eventual results by helping the surgeon determine when adequate surgery has been performed.

The patient is anesthetized with topical proparacaine hydrochloride. The periocular skin is prepped utilizing a povidone/iodine solution. A sterile field is achieved with a plastic adhesive aperture drape and the lids are separated with a fine wire speculum. The patient is asked to fixate the operating microscope light and the keratometer mire is studied on the corneal surface. The axis of the steepest meridian is noted and a mark is made with a blade in the epithelium on each side of the graft host interface (Figure 11-1). The appropriate incision length is approximately 60° to 90° or 15% to 25% of the circumference of the graft. The incision length and depth should vary depending on the type of wound healing that has yielded the astigmatism. Utilization of intraoperative keratometry is especially useful during performance of the relaxing incision. The length and depth of the incisions can be graded according to the effect achieved during the surgical procedure.

We prefer to carefully dissect in the graft-host interface in a graded fashion utilizing a micro-sharp metal blade (Figure 11-2). This technique allows us to gently scratch down into the incision while continuously observing the keratometer mire for correction of the astigmatism. As wound healing is quite variable in the graft host interface in keratoplasty patients, it is not unusual to enter areas of poor wound healing. In such cases the incision can be more carefully titrated and adjusted utilizing this

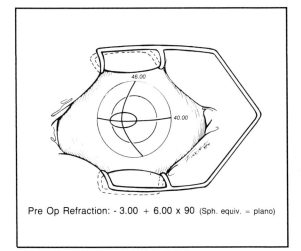

Pre Op Refraction: - 3.00 + 6.00 x 90 (Sph. equiv. = plano)

Figure 11-1. Relaxing incision.

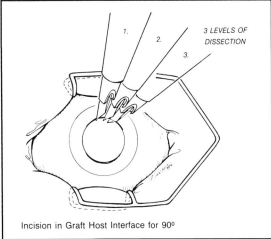

3 LEVELS OF DISSECTION

Incision in Graft Host Interface for 90º

Figure 11-2. Relaxing incision.

technique. We have attempted the use of preset diamond knives as used in radial keratotomy; however, we found that in many instances we either caused perforations or were unable to maintain the incision in the graft-host interface because of poor visibility. In addition, the slow and careful deepening of the incision appears to be more controllable in our hands with the metal knife than with the nonguarded diamond knife. In some cases we actually resort to blunt dissection with the noncutting edge of the knife. If perforation occurs with significant loss of chamber, suturing is necessary. Unfortunately, this suturing usually negates any effect of the operation. Occasionally early removal of the suture (four to six weeks) will still allow for some effect.

Progressive deepening and lengthening of the incision is performed first on one side and then on the other side until an overcorrection is achieved according to observation of the keratometer mires. In general, we expect to lose approximately one-third to one-half of the effect of the surgery during postoperative healing, and therefore we try to overcorrect the patient 30-50% of their preoperative cylinder. For example, if the preoperative cylinder is 6 diopters we will try to achieve a 2 to 3 diopter overcorrection.

Compression Sutures. If a satisfactory correction cannot be obtained utilizing the simple relaxing incision technique, two 10-0 prolene compression sutures are placed on each side of the graft-host interface 90° away from the relaxing incision (Figure 11-3). These sutures are tied with a simple slip knot and tightened under keratometric control until appropriate overcorrection is achieved (Figure 11-4). The knots are then cut short and buried. We prefer to utilize prolene sutures since, in some cases, a perfect surgical correction of the astigmatism is achieved and it is desirable to leave the suture in for extended periods of time. Nylon will hydrolyze in one to two years whereas the prolene will last as long as seven to 10 years.

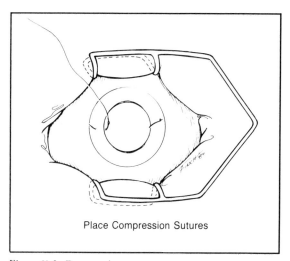

Place Compression Sutures

Figure 11-3. Compression suture.

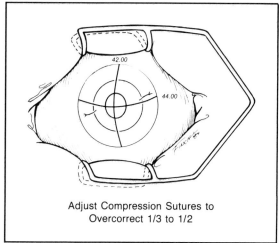

Adjust Compression Sutures to
Overcorrect 1/3 to 1/2

Figure 11-4. Compression suture.

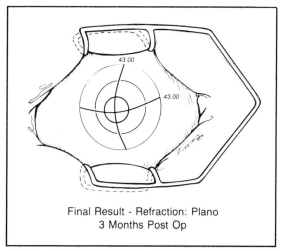

Final Result - Refraction: Plano
3 Months Post Op

Figure 11-5. Compression suture.

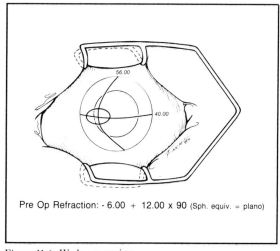

Pre Op Refraction: - 6.00 + 12.00 x 90 (Sph. equiv. = plano)

Figure 11-6. Wedge resection

After completion of surgery, the relaxing incisions are gently irrigated with a blunt cannula to remove any blood or debris. The globe is irrigated with topical gentamicin sulfate. In most cases a single drop of 0.25% scopolamine hydrochloride is placed on the eye for cycloplegia. The eye is covered with a patch and shield. The patient is asked to return the following day for evaluation.

Postoperative Course. Postoperatively the patient is treated with topical antibiotics four times daily for one week. Topical steroids are continued as appropriate for maintenance of graft clarity. Serial keratometry and refraction are performed and when the eye is stable, optical correction is provided with glasses or contact lens (Figure 11-5).

If compression sutures have been utilized and overcorrection persists at eight weeks, one of the sutures is removed. The patient is asked to return, and if overcorrection still persists, the second compression suture is removed at 12 weeks. If an inadequate surgical correction is achieved, the operation may be repeated or an alternative procedure such as wedge resection, compression suture technique, or astigmatic keratotomy may be considered.

Wedge Resection

Introduction. The wedge resection technique for correction of post-keratoplasty astigmatism is appropriate for cases with relatively high levels of cylinder.[1,3-7] This technique is capable of correcting up to 20 diopters of astigmatism. We currently prefer to attempt to correct most cases with astigmatism less than 10 to 15 diopters by using relaxing incisions or astigmatic keratotomy prior to considering wedge resection. The wedge resection approach requires a longer postoperative visual rehabilitation. The longer visual rehabilitation is needed because the multiple sutures induce significant irregular astigmatism and wound healing must take place with selective suture removal to reduce the astigmatism prior to eventual visual rehabilitation. Nonetheless, the alternative to this procedure in patients with severe astigmatism is consideration of repeat keratoplasty. The wedge resection approach should always be attempted first.

Operative Technique. The patient is evaluated preoperatively as described for the relaxing incision. We have found that the overall effect of the wedge resection is to steepen the flatter meridian approximately twice as much as it flattens the steeper meridian. This effect means that the average patient will have a slight increase in myopia or decrease in hyperopia following this surgical technique. For example, if the preoperative refraction and keratometry readings were -6.00 $+12.00$ $\times 90$ ($+6.00$ -6.00 $\times 180$) and the keratometry readings $40.00/52.00$ $\times 90$ and we obtain a perfect result, we expect our postoperative results to be a keratometry reading of $48.00/48.00$ with a refraction of -2 diopters. This is a 2 diopter myopic shift.

A wedge resection requires retrobulbar anesthesia as the dissection of the wedge resection and placement of the multiple sutures requires good akinesia. To begin, the axis of the flattest meridian is marked, preferably under intraoperative surgical control with an operating keratometer (Figure 11-6). In the wedge resection technique a diamond micrometer radial keratotomy knife is useful. If a double-bladed knife as described by Troutman is available, it can be utilized but we have not had access to the instrument.[5] In addition, intraoperative ultrasonic pachymetry is helpful.

Ultrasonic pachymetry is performed at the graft-host interface in the axis where the wedge resection is to be performed. It is usually impossible to obtain readings immediately over the scar; however, readings can commonly be obtained adjacent to the graft-host interface just onto the donor or recipient. Several corneal thickness measurements are taken and the diamond knife is set at 100% of the thinnest reading. The blade setting is then checked with a coin gauge or similar device. A 90° section of the keratoplasty wound is then incised with the diamond knife. An attempt is made to stay in the graft-host interface but perfect accuracy is difficult. A wedge of recipient tissue is then excised with the diamond knife utilizing a free hand dissection (Figure 11-7).

In the average case resection of a tenth of a millimeter of tissue results in approximately 2 diopters of correction. We reserve this operation for patients with greater than 10 diopters of astigmatism and therefore resect on the average 0.5 to 1 mm of tissue. We have not found it necessary to perform a paracentesis prior to resuturing this wound. We then place five to seven deep evenly-spaced interrupted 10-0 prolene sutures (Figure 11-8). Once again we prefer prolene sutures as this allows us to leave the sutures in place indefinitely if desirable. Each of the sutures is placed with a slip knot and, under keratometric control, the sutures are tightened until an overcorrection of one-third to one-half of the preoperative cylinder is achieved (Figure 11-9). For example, if the preoperative astigmatism was 12 diopters, we will tighten the sutures until a 4 to 6 diopter astigmatism is achieved in the axis opposite to the preoperative cylinder. The sutures are then tied down with square knots, cut short and buried.

Postoperative Course. The immediate postoperative care is the same as that for relaxing incisions. The sutures are left in place for a minimum of eight weeks. At eight weeks a selective suture removal technique in the axis of the steepest residual astigmatism is utilized with one to two sutures being removed every three to four weeks. Once a satisfactory result is achieved the remaining sutures may be left indefinitely, particularly if prolene is utilized (Figure 11-10).

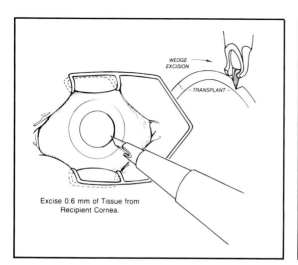

Figure 11-7. Wedge resection

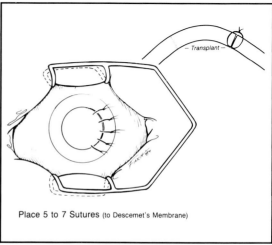

Figure 11-8. Wedge resection

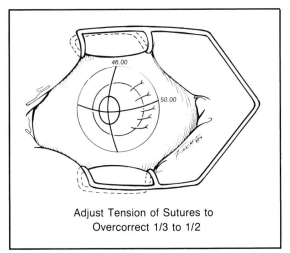

Adjust Tension of Sutures to
Overcorrect 1/3 to 1/2

Figure 11-9. Wedge resection

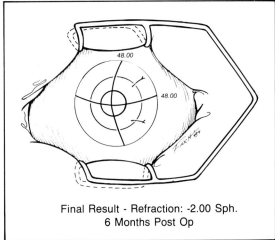

Final Result - Refraction: -2.00 Sph.
6 Months Post Op

Figure 11-10. Wedge resection

Wound Revision/Compression Suture

Introduction. We have found the wound revision/compression suture technique to be useful in some cases of post-keratoplasty astigmatism. This technique is essentially a hybrid of the relaxing incision and wedge resection. In particular, this approach may be attempted in cases where relaxing incision has been performed and there is significant undercorrection. Preoperative evaluation is done as previously described. The essential pattern of refractive change is similar to that obtained in the relaxing incision.

Technique. Retrobulbar anesthesia is again preferred and the flat meridian is marked (Figure 11-11). A dissection to three-fourths to seven-eighths depth is made in the keratoplasty incision in the flatter meridian. This dissection is identical in regards to incision making technique as that utilized for the relaxing incision (Figure 11-12). The remainder of the operation is identical to that described in the wedge resection technique except that no tissue is excised. We simply place five to seven deep evenly spaced interrupted 10-0 prolene sutures and adjust their tension with the surgical keratometer to achieve a one-third to one-half overcorrection of the preexisting astigmatism (Figure 11-13). The sutures are then removed selectively postoperatively beginning at two months as in the wedge resection technique in order to attempt to reduce residual astigmatism (Figure 11-14).

We have found this technique useful for correcting as much as 4 to 6 diopters of residual astigmatism following relaxing incision when a repeat of the relaxing incision was not felt prudent and wedge resection was expected to produce an overcorrection.

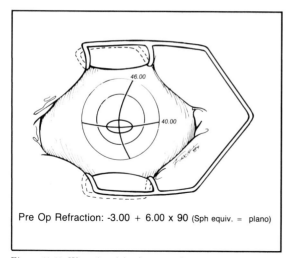

Pre Op Refraction: -3.00 + 6.00 x 90 (Sph equiv. = plano)

Figure 11-11. Wound revision/compression suture.

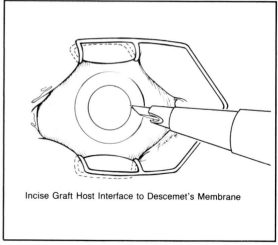

Incise Graft Host Interface to Descemet's Membrane

Figure 11-12. Wound revision/compression suture.

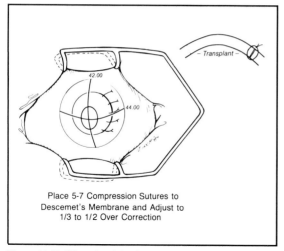

Place 5-7 Compression Sutures to
Descemet's Membrane and Adjust to
1/3 to 1/2 Over Correction

Figure 11-13. Wound revision/compression suture.

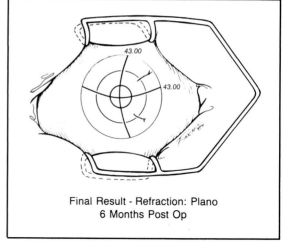

Final Result - Refraction: Plano
6 Months Post Op

Figure 11-14. Wound revision/compression suture.

Astigmatic Keratotomy

Introduction. A large number of techniques based on the radial keratotomy approach for the correction of astigmatism have evolved.[8-10] We
have found two techniques to be particularly useful for the correction of
postoperative astigmatism. One technique is the use of simple tangential
incisions 4.0 mm in length for the correction of low degrees of astigmatism.
The other technique is the Ruiz astigmatic keratotomy for the correction of

moderate to high amounts of astigmatism (2.50 to 12.0 diopters of astigmatism).

We have found that one or two tangential incisions at an optical zone of 4 to 6 mm with a length of 2.5 mm can correct 2 to 4 diopters of astigmatism (Figures 11-15, 11-16, 11-17). The Ruiz astigmatic keratotomy utilizes a combination of four tangential incisions combined with four radial incisions. This technique allows selection of variable optical clear zone diameters and therefore the operation can be graded. We have found that the amount of astigmatism corrected is dependent on the clear zone and the depth of the incisions.[10] We have preferred to use deep incisions with a larger clear zone, and therefore we utilize intraoperative ultrasonic pachymetry to set a guarded diamond knife for the procedure. The amount of astigmatism which can be corrected depends also on multiple other factors such as age as previously noted in radial keratotomy research. We have, however, found that we can correct from 2 diopters to as much as 12 diopters in some older patients with this procedure. The operation also has the advantage of being gradable by varying the optical zone.

Operative Technique. The techniques for the tangential incisions and Ruiz astigmatic keratotomy are similar to those utilized for radial keratotomy. The patient is evaluated preoperatively with refraction, keratometry, and corneoscopy. We find that the tangential incisions tend to produce minimal change in the overall spherical equivalent of the eye, acting similar to a relaxing incision. The Ruiz procedure, on the other hand, results in significant overall mean flattening of the cornea and therefore reduces myopia or increases hyperopia. The ratio of flattening of the steeper meridian to steeping of the flatter meridian in the Ruiz procedure depends on the length of the tangential incisions and the size of the optical zone. On the average, the flattening:steepening ratio appears to be in the range of 5:1 or 6:1 when utilizing a 2.5 mm length tangential

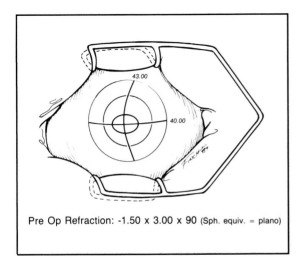

Pre Op Refraction: -1.50 x 3.00 x 90 (Sph. equiv. = plano)

Figure 11-15. Tangential incisions.

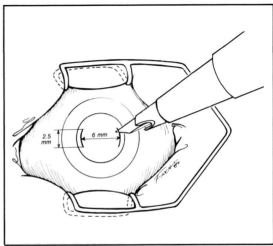

Figure 11-16. Tangential incisions.

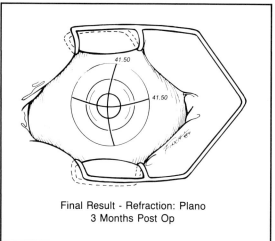

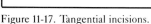

Final Result - Refraction: Plano
3 Months Post Op

Figure 11-17. Tangential incisions.

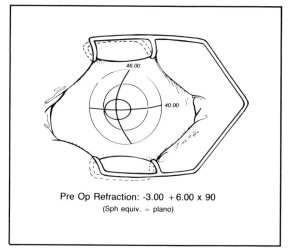

Pre Op Refraction: -3.00 +6.00 x 90
(Sph equiv. = plano)

Figure 11-18. Ruiz procedure.

stepladder incision. This means that if our theoretical patient with a preoperative refractive error of $-3.00 +6.00 \times 90$ and keratometry readings of $40.00/46.00 \times 90$ were operated with a Ruiz astigmatic keratotomy and achieved a perfect result, we would expect a postoperative keratometry of approximately 41.00/41.00 and a postoperative refraction of +2.00 sphere. This is the opposite result to that achieved with a wedge resection. Thus it is important in some cases for the surgeon to select the appropriate operation to correct or reduce induced ametropia. It must be stated that these techniques are currently in a state of rapid evolution and minimal solid data is available to evaluate safety and efficacy. The following is the current approach utilized in our clinic.

Operative Technique. The patient is operated upon utilizing an operating microscope and a surgical keratometer (Figure 11-18). The preparation is the same as for the relaxing incision. Topical anesthesia is adequate for these cases. The patient's preoperative corneal diameter is measured and noted for future reference. The patient is asked to fixate the operating microscope. While the surgeon looks through the right eye piece with the left eye closed, a small mark is placed at the left inferior edge of the reflection of the microscope light filament (Figure 11-19). The appropriate optical zone marker is then selected and, using the cross hairs centered on the visual axis, mild pressure is applied and a ring mark on the epithelium is created (Figure 11-20). The eye is then moistened with Balanced Salt Solution and, using an ultrasonic pachymeter, central corneal thickness and corneal thickness in the axis of the steep corneal merdian adjacent to the optical zone marker are measured (Figure 11-21). An adjustable micrometer diamond knife is set to full depth of the thinnest paracentral ultrasonic corneal pachymetry reading (Figure 11-22). The blade depth is checked on a depth gauge and adjusted appropriately for accuracy (Figure 11-23). If single tangential incisions are to be placed for correction of small amounts of astigmatism, we prefer a 5 mm to 6 mm optical zone. If more correction is preferred, the Ruiz astigmatic keratotomy is selected with a 3 mm to 6 mm optical zone. We prefer not to use smaller than a 3 mm optical zone. In general the amount of correction expected with the Ruiz astigmatic keratotomy for each optical zone and depth of cut is noted in Table 11-1. This table has been adapted from reports by Luis Ruiz and is only a general approximation. We find, for example, a significant variation in the effect in younger versus older patients and a somewhat variable effect in post-keratoplasty patients. Further experience is needed in this operation to improve predictability and assess potential adverse side effects.

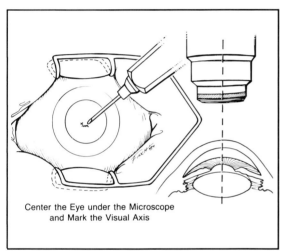

Center the Eye under the Microscope
and Mark the Visual Axis

Figure 11-19. Ruiz procedure.

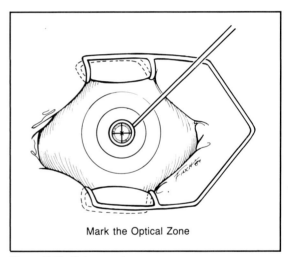

Mark the Optical Zone

Figure 11-20. Ruiz procedure.

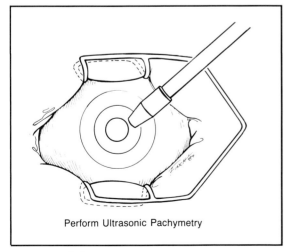

Perform Ultrasonic Pachymetry

Figure 11-21. Ruiz procedure.

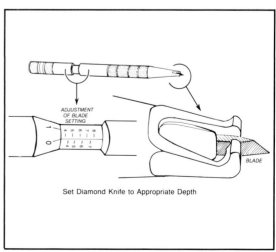

ADJUSTMENT
OF BLADE
SETTING

BLADE

Set Diamond Knife to Appropriate Depth

Figure 11-22. Ruiz procedure.

TABLE 11-1

Modified Ruiz Technique - Correction of Astigmatism
Four cuts - 2.5 mm in length with radial incisions

OPTICAL CLEAR ZONE										
5.0	0.50	0.75	1.00	1.25	1.50	1.75	2.00	2.25	2.50	2.75
4.5	1.00	1.50	2.00	2.50	3.00	3.50	4.00	4.50	5.00	5.50
4.4	1.50	2.25	3.00	3.75	4.50	5.25	6.00	6.75	7.50	8.25
3.5	2.00	3.00	4.00	5.00	6.00	7.00	8.00	9.00	10.00	11.00
3.0	2.50	3.75	5.00	6.25	7.50	8.75	10.00	11.25	12.50	13.75
	40%	50%	60%	70%	80%	90%	100%	110%	120%	130%

Blade Depth as Percent of Central Corneal Thickness

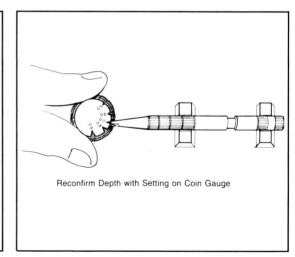

Reconfirm Depth with Setting on Coin Gauge

Figure 11-23. Ruiz procedure.

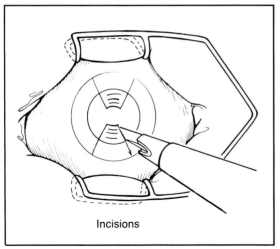

Incisions

Figure 11-24. Ruiz procedure.

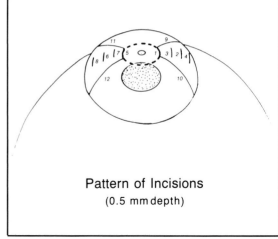

Pattern of Incisions
(0.5 mm depth)

Figure 11-25. Ruiz procedure.

For simple tangential astigmatic keratotomy a 4.0 mm incision is made tangential to the optical zone mark (Figure 11-24). The globe is fixated and the diamond knife is inserted into the cornea perpendicular to the surface. A 1 to 2 second hesitation is preferred, prior to beginning the cut to allow settling of the blade; then a slow purposeful incision toward the radial incision is made for an extent of 4.0 mm. The knife is then removed and a similar incision made on the opposite side toward the radial incision to avoid lamellar stromal dehiscence. In most cases an immediate rounding of the keratometer mire is noted on the surgical keratometer (Figure 11-25). If inadequate correction is noted, a second tangential incision may be made approximately 1 mm inside or outside the first incision.

For the Ruiz astigmatic keratotomy a similar tangential incision is made on each side of the optical zone marker. A second tangential incision is made halfway between the initial tangential incision and the limbus and two additional tangential incisions are made between the first two incisions and between the second incision and the limbus. This creates four stepladder tangential incisions on each side of the optical zone in the axis of the steeper merdiain.

Four radial incisions are then made in the following fashion. The knife blade is placed in the lateral extent of the innermost tangential incision. The radial incision should be made such that its course is halfway between the radial and perpendicular to the tangential incision. We do this by sighting the center of the cornea and determining mentally what a radial incision would be and comparing this with an incision that would be perpendicular to the edge of each of the tangential incisions. The preferred angle of the radial incision is then halfway between these two imaginary lines. Four radial incisions are then completed, stopping inside the paralimbal vascular arcade to avoid bleeding.

The incisions are gently irrigated with a 25 to 30 gauge cannula using Balanced Salt Solution to remove any blood or debris (Figures 11-26 and 11-27). The globe is irrigated with gentamicin and a drop of topical 0.25% scopolamine hydrochloride placed on the eye as in the relaxing incision technique. In post-keratoplasty cases a patch and shield are placed on the post-keratoplasty cases a patch and shield are placed on the eye.

Postoperative care includes topical antibiotics four times daily for one week. Steroids may be used as needed for maintenance of graft clarity or to control inflammation. It is possible that a slightly greater effect may be achieved through the utilization of topical steroids. If early postoperative

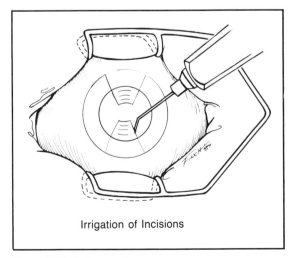

Irrigation of Incisions

Figure 11-26. Ruiz procedure.

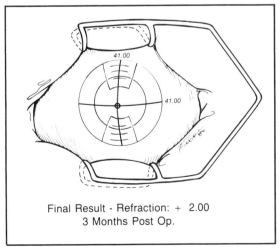

Final Result - Refraction: + 2.00
3 Months Post Op.

Figure 11-27. Ruiz procedure.

readings suggest undercorrection, topical steroids may be applied four times daily for six to eight weeks.

The techniques for surgical correction of postoperative astigmatism are currently in evolution and considerable attention will be directed to the technique of astigmatic keratotomy in coming years. It is expected that the above techniques will prove useful and it is certain that the surgical techniques described will evolve. In addition, it is expected that new techniques will be developed in the near future. It is hoped that the above descriptions will prove useful and be adaptable to other surgeons who care for such difficult patients.

References

1. Troutman RC: *Microsurgery of the Anterior Segment of the Eye*, Vol 2. St Louis: CV Mosby, p 286, 1977.
2. Troutman RC, Swinger C: Relaxing Incision for Control of Postoperative Astigmatism Following Keratoplasty. *Ophthal Surg* 11:117-120, 1980.
3. Krachmer JH, Fenzl RE: Surgical Correction of High Postkeratoplasty Astigmatism. *Arch Ophthalmol* 98:1400-1402, 1980.
4. Krachmer JH, Ching SST: Relaxing Corneal Incisions for Postkeratoplasty Astigmatism. *Int Ophthalmol Clin* 23(4):153-157, 1983.
5. Troutman RC: Corneal Wedge Resections and Relaxing Incisions for Postkeratoplasty Astigmatism. *Int Ophthalmol Clin* 23(4):161-168, 1983.
6. Lavery GW, Lindstrom RL, Hofer LA, Doughman DJ: The Surgical Management of Corneal Astigmatism after Penetrating Keratoplasty (Submitted, *Ophthal Surg*).
7. Barner SS: Surgical Treatment of Corneal Astigmatism. *Ophthal Surg* 7:43-48, 1976.
8. Sanders D: *Radial Keratotomy: ARK Study Group,* Thorofare, NJ: Slack, Inc., 1984.
9. Nordan LT: *Current Status of Refractive Surgery.* San Diego, CA: Lee T. Nordan, MD, 1983.
10. Lavery GW, Lindstrom RL: Astigmatic Keratotomy in Human Cadaver Eyes (Submitted, *Cornea*).

Chapter 12

Postoperative Management
Robert F. Hofmann, MD

POSTOPERATIVE MANAGEMENT

In radial keratotomy, the routine postoperative management in an uncomplicated case is relatively simple. The time course of the transient side effects of the surgery is somewhat predictable and reassuring. It is difficult for the surgeon to cause an unfortunate long-term result due to faulty postoperative care. Nevertheless, a few basic principles should be discussed in order to provide guidelines for the postoperative care of the patient who has undergone incisional refractive keratoplasty.

Wound Irrigation

Immediately upon completion of the corneal incisions the eye should be checked for correct incisional depths, and the wounds should be irrigated with balanced salt solution. All blood, epithelial cells,[1] and debris should be vigorously irrigated without spreading or stretching the corneal lamellae. The inclusions of epithelium and blood will not affect the optical outcome of the surgery; however, these inclusions are disheartening to the surgeon at slit lamp examination postoperatively. Inclusions into the incisions often extrude with time, but they may be present for future surgeons to see in the patient's cornea for years to come.

Bandaging

There is a mild controversy[2] as to whether the eyes should be patched, steri-stripped or left alone during the immediate postoperative period. The advocates of the open eye approach feel that patching does not significantly enhance re-epithelialization over the incisions. They also feel that the patient has the same postoperative foreign body sensation with or without a patch. Some advocates of avoiding patching also feel that a warm humid environment which is excellent for culturing bacteria exists under a compression patch. The advocates of patching would state that it is better to protect the eye from inadvertent placement of foreign bodies in the immediate postoperative period with a patch. They also feel that with a moderately tight double pressure patch the eye is in contact with mucosal surfaces which would make the patient more comfortable. The steri-strip advocates would include the benefits from both of the previous points of view. Regardless of the early postoperative protection, the key point is that the patient be kept away from particulate, biological, or toxic matter which could enter the incisions prior to re-epithelialization.

Antibiotics

Postoperative antibiotics can be administered subconjunctivally, topically, orally, or parenterally. The immediate postoperative use of subconjunctival injection of antibiotics should be tempered by the postoperative pain and subconjunctival hemorrhaging which frequently occur with this modality. The patient operated under topical anesthesia does not have sufficient anesthesia for painless subconjunctival injection. Perhaps the subconjunctival route is best applied to those cases in which there is actual perforation into the anterior chamber during surgery. The topical application of antibiotics will decrease the colony counts but will not sterilize the cornea. Copious irrigation of the corneal surface prior to application of the patch probably is of some benefit in decreasing the innoculum of bacteria. Parenteral and oral antibiotics would not provide a significant enhancement of local levels of antibiotics and would be of little use in these patients. Ointments should not be applied in the postoperative incisional refractive keratoplasty eye due to the fact that white petrolatum, mineral oil, and other petroleum distillates can find their way into the depth of the incisions. The choice of topical antibiotic drops is left solely to the discretion of the individual surgeon. The guidelines for prophylaxis postoperatively are that the antibiotics have sufficient broad spectrum of coverage with limited toxicity either systemically or locally. The separation of antibiotics from steroids is preferred in that the antibiotics can be discontinued within four to five days postoperatively once re-epithelialization has occurred. The continuation of epithelial toxic antibiotics such as neomycin, gentamicin or tobramycin may actually induce punctate epithelial keratopathy on a toxic or allergic basis. The excessive use of potent broad spectrum antibiotics can induce complications such as keratoconjunctivitis, allergy, bone marrow depression and a selection of fungal species.

Steroids

Topical corticosteroids provide both beneficial and harmful effects[3] upon the healing of the radial keratotomy wound. Immediately postoperatively the corneal stroma and epithelium swell for 24 to 36 hours due to the effect of the incisions alone. The average postoperative overcorrection on day one which can be generally expected in an eight-incision radial keratotomy is approximately 2.00 diopters; 1.50 diopters in a four-incision; and 2.50 diopters in a 16-incision radial keratotomy. This effect is expected and is not generally influenced by the use of steroids. Early use of steroids prior to prompt epithelialization of the incisions can be deleterious especially in patients who are exposed to a significant biological innoculum.[4] Topical steroid medications are frequently used by surgeons to decrease postoperative iritis, conjunctival injection, pain, and to reduce an overly rapid regression of surgical effect. Immediate reduction in regression by the use of steroids can be related to the secondary rise in intraocular pressure which causes central flattening of the cornea. This steroid effect can only be used temporarily for a few weeks and should not be used long term because of the chance of a steroid-induced glaucoma or cataracts. The hope of using steroid medication to prevent collagen formation and cross linking is not feasible because of the steroids' ineffectiveness and long-term side effects of topical steroids upon the eye.[3,4]

Analgesia

The postoperative pain incurred by the patient is generally of a mild to moderate nature, mostly being a foreign body sensation. It is very rare for a patient to have severe postoperative pain unless the case has been extremely prolonged, incisions have crossed the limbus, or the patient has a low threshold to pain. Most of the discomfort is due to a foreign body sensation from the baring of nerve endings at the incisional sites. This foreign body sensation is generally most severe for approximately four to five hours postoperatively under topical anesthesia and will last to a mild degree for approximately two to three days. Extremely strong narcotic medications are probably not necessary for radial keratotomy patients and may actually induce more nausea and discomfort. Sedatives given postoperatively should be mild and for only a few doses to allow the patient to sleep comfortably for the first night. Adequate pain control can be accomplished simply by the application of a cold wet compress to the lids combined with Motrin 600 mg given preoperatively and immediately postoperatively. The deep ciliary pain is due to cyclospasm and possibly the release of prostaglandins from the iris. The prostaglandin synthetase inhibitors may moderate this effect. Cycloplegic agents are used by some surgeons to decrease the immediate postoperative ciliary pain and photophobia. Care must be taken that short to intermediate acting agents alone are used. The use of atropine or scopolamine should be discouraged because the persistent dilatation of the pupil induces more glare and visual discomfort to the patient than the mild postoperative iritis. With the more modern approach of keeping the incisions within the cornea itself and with the decrease in emphasis on re-deepening procedures in the periphery,[5] there is a significant drop in postoperative pain.

Restrictions

The postoperative restrictions placed upon the incisional refractive keratoplasty patient are actually quite bearable. The patient needs to understand that he should avoid any ocular trauma, exposure to toxic agents, or innoculation by bacterial substances. The patient must be encouraged to keep his eye well lubricated during the first three to five days postoperatively when epithelialization is taking place. Artificial tears and lubricant ointments are frequently required for the first month because of a nonspecific punctate keratopathy from surface distortion with local wetting defects. Women should be discouraged from wearing eyeliners or mascara as the introduction of foreign material from the lashline could be a source of contamination and infection. Showering should be accomplished with the eye protected from direct application of water or soap. A Fox metal shield should be encouraged at bedtime for use in the first week postoperatively because many patients inadvertently will rub their eyes at night. Since the anterior chamber is not entered at surgery in an uncomplicated case, the patient theoretically need not worry about bending, stooping, or lifting. The patient can sleep on either side and lift normal amounts for work. Smoking is to be discouraged as is exposure to any toxic fume or substance. Hard contact sports are to be discouraged for at least six months to a year and polycarbonate protective eye wear for sports such as racquetball, squash, and tennis is to be mandated. Water sports such as scuba diving should be discouraged for a few months and the patient should be instructed that there will be significant fluctuations in visual acuity dependent upon the atmospheric pressure at high altitudes or water pressure at low depths.

Glare Protection

Since transient glare is of an unpredictable nature, the patient should be offered the use of polarizing or darkly tinted sunglasses. With the advent of the four- and six-incision radial keratotomy, some patients may not need any protection from sunlight. With the 12- and 16-incision radial keratotomies, glare can be significant, prolonged, and cause discomfort. Immediately postoperatively both for the patient's protection and the surgeon's medicolegal protection the patient should be instructed to avoid night driving as long as the glare is significant. There have been some patients who have had motor vehicle accidents within a few evenings of a radial keratotomy.

Contact Lenses

Corneal neovascularization induced by contact lenses follows a number of proposed mechanisms. Inflammatory mediators, hypoxia, mechanical trauma, plastic toxicity, and stromal edema have all been implicated as inciting agents.[6-10] Although uncomplicated radial keratotomy has not been related to corneal neovascularization, the addition of contact lenses of any type in the healing phase (one year) has caused corneal neovascularization. This postoperative contact lens induced neovascularization has been seen with daily wear, extended wear, hard and gas-permeable lenses in both laboratory and clinical situations. Although approximately 20% of radial keratotomy patients require residual correction, contact lenses should be considered very late and with close follow-up. Remember—the patient had the surgery to get away from prosthetic optical devices. The surgeon should re-evaluate his motivations, plan, and procedure if he is getting a number of patients miscorrected enough to even consider a postoperative contact lens.

Besides the neovascularization risk, the post-radial keratotomy cornea is difficult to fit with a contact lens and may be impossible.[11] Postoperative orthokeratology to modify surgical results has limited theoretical appeal and, except for a few anecdotal oral reports, has not been reported in a controlled study in the literature to date.

Effect Enhancement

The response of the human cornea to controlled radial keratotomy surgical trauma is not unlike its response to other forms of incisional trauma.[12] The acute inflammatory reaction initially causes the wound to swell for the first 24 to 48 hours. As the acute inflammatory reaction subsides, the epithelium slides across the superficial defect. Myofibroblastic cells have not been demonstrated histologically in radial keratotomy specimens.[13,14] The initial reduction in flattening over the first week post-radial keratotomy is probably due to the resolution of the acute inflammatory response. The long-term regression phase from three weeks to six months is characterized by the deposition and cross-linking of collagen at the wound site. This long-term extracellular phase leads to wound contraction and scar formation.

Collagen cross-linking is mediated by the copper-dependent enzyme lysyl oxidase. The extract of the fava bean, Beta-aminoproprionitrile is known to be a powerful inhibitor of the cross-linking enzyme lysyl oxidase.[15,16,17] This compound has been used for the control of esophageal, bladder, sphincter, and flexor tendon cicatrization in both humans and experimental animals. In these applications, the drug was given systemically and had some undesirable aspects such as periosteal reaction and rash. Beta-aminoproprionitrile has met with some success when applied topically to keloids and peritendinous adhesions in animals. Moorhead has had some success with its topical application in limiting fornix contracture after alkali burns of the conjunctiva in rabbits.[18] It also has been shown in rabbits to decrease the extent of vitreous proliferation following perforating injury.[19] Its recent experimental use in rabbits as 33% (wt) in petrolatum under controlled conditions following radial keratotomy by both Moorhead[15] and Kogan, et al[16] in separate studies has indicated an approximate 20% enhancement of the surgical effect of radial keratotomy. These published studies by separate groups indicate a means for the future of potentially undoing the regression due to long-term extracellular collagen cross-linking. Controlled human studies are under way but as yet, no conclusions have been determined long term. The potential, however, for reducing collagen contracture and enhancing surgical effect in a reliable manner may decrease the incidence of surgical undercorrection.

Drugs such as Prostaglandin E_1 and Beta-phenylethylamine increase effect by increasing intraocular pressure. However, these drugs are not wound healing, increase corneal instability, and prolong visual fluctuation. Steroids do *not* have a long-term benefit upon effect enhancement and, thus, are not recommended for use beyond a few weeks postoperatively to decrease initial inflammation.

clinically available and can cause intraocular inflammation. Corticosteroids are unpredictable in their effect on intraocular pressure, and they retard

Regression Enhancement

Just as pharmacologic means for reducing regression are being introduced, there are standard means presently available to reduce an overcorrection in radial keratotomy. Although there is not presently available a drug to enhance fibroblast proliferation or collagen cross-linking, the parameter of intraocular pressure can be controlled during corneal healing. When the pressure inside the corneal dome, which has been weakened by peripheral cuts, is lessened, then the central curvature of the dome is steepened. Antiglaucoma therapy can be utilized to perform this manipulation. Although in general antiglaucoma medications do not lower intraocular pressure very much in normotensive eyes, even a small decrement can reduce hyperopia. The use of 0.5% or 1% pilocarpine, for instance, may have multiple positive effects. The miotics induce transient myopia, increased depth of focus through pupillary constriction, and reduction in intraocular pressure. All three of these effects can reduce hyperopia and improve the quality of visual image, especially in a glare-induced situation. The untoward effect of strong miotics such as ciliary pain, dimming of vision and excessive myopia balance the potential positive effects of these drugs.

Timolol maleate 0.5% can be applied twice each day for pressure reduction without the side effect of miosis. This drug is used routinely with minimal side effects in multiple forms of glaucoma, and for the most part can be applied safely in the post-radial keratotomy patient. Nevertheless, the side effects of increased foreign body sensation, dry eye sensation, punctate keratopathy and the systemic effects in asthmatics must be borne in mind by the clinician. The epinephrine analog drugs require a loading time measured in weeks which would tend to reduce their effectiveness in modulating the overcorrection of a radial keratotomy patient. Carbonic anhydrase inhibitors lower intraocular pressure effectively but their side effects (GI disturbance, electrolyte imbalance, renal stones, paresthesias, etc.) negate their usefulness long term in refractive surgery. Marijuana is a commonly used hallucinogen in our society which lowers intraocular pressure and increases regression of radial keratotomy effect. It can *not* ethically be recommended as a drug by the surgeon, but must be considered as a potential agent in excessive regression with low intraocular pressure in the face of well executed radial keratotomy.

Conclusion

The routine postoperative management of the radial keratotomy patient is decidedly simple. The transient effects of glare, mild punctate keratopathy, foreign body sensation, and mild iritis need minimal treatment. With common sense and a good clinical and pharmacological acumen, the uncomplicated radial keratotomy patient can be managed with very few drugs or manipulations. When combined with appropriate preoperative counseling, the postoperative course of the refractive keratoplasty patient can be extremely smooth. Lack of attention to the basic mechanics of corneal wound healing and the corneal immune barriers results in some instances in potentially disastrous complications in a previously virgin cornea.

References

1. Jester J, Villaseñor RA, Miyashiro J: Epithelial Inclusion Cysts Following Radial Keratotomy. *Arch Ophthalmol* 101:611-615, 1983.
2. Sanders, DR: *Radial Keratotomy: ARK Study Group.* Thorofare, NJ: Slack Inc., 1984, p 92.
3. Yamaguchi T, Asbell PA, Ostrick M, et al.: Corticosteroid Therapy after Anterior Radial Keratotomy in Primates. *Am J Ophthalmol* 97:215-220, 1984.
4. Kaufman HE: Practical Considerations in the Selection of Anti-inflammatory Agents. *Trans Am Acad Ophthalmol Otolaryngol* 79:OP-89, 1975.
5. Schachar RA, Black TD, Huang T: *Understanding Radial Keratotomy.* Dennison, TX: LAL Publishing, 1981, pp 52-65.
6. Binder PS: Complications Associated with Extended-wear Soft Contact Lenses. *Ophthalmology* 86:1093, 1979.
7. Nesburn A: Complications Associated with Therapeutic Soft Contact Lenses. *Ophthalmology* 86:1130, 1978.
8. Kaufman HE: Problems Associated with Prolonged-wear Soft Contact Lenses. *Ophthalmology* 86:441, 1978.
9. Dixon JM, Lawaczek E: Corneal Neovascularization Due to Contact Lenses. *Arch Ophthalmol* 69:72, 1963.
10. Federman JL, Brown GC, Felberg NT: Experimental Ocular Angiogenesis. *Am J Ophthalmol* 89:231, 1980.
11. Rowsey JJ, Balyeat HD: Preliminary Results and Complications of Radial Keratotomy. *Am J Ophthalmol* 93:437, 1982.
12. Kurasova TP: Clinical Course of the Postoperative Period after Keratotomy. *Surgery of Anomalies of Eye Refraction.* Moscow, 1981.
13. Schachar RA, Black TD, Huang T: *Understanding Radial Keratotomy.* Dennison, TX: LAL Publishing, 1981, pp 79-99.
14. Stainer GA, Shaw EL, Binder PS: Histopathology of a Case of Radial Keratotomy. *Arch Ophthalmol* 100:1473-1477, 1982.
15. Moorhead LC, Carroll J, Constance G: Effects of Topical Treatment with Beta-aminoproprionitrite after Radial Keratotomy in the Rabbit. *Arch Ophthalmol* 102:304-307, 1984.
16. Kogan LL, Katzen L: Enhancement of Radial Keratotomy by Chemical Inhibition of Collagen Cross-linkages: A preliminary report. *Ann Ophthalmol* 15:842-845, 1983.
17. Siegel RC, Martin AR: Collagen Cross-linking: Enzymatic synthesis of lysine-derived aldehydes and the production of cross-linked components. *J Biol Chem* 245:1653-1658, 1970.
18. Moorhead LC: Inhibition of Collagen Cross-linking: A new approach to ocular scarring. *Curr Eye Res* 9:77-83, 1981.
19. Moorhead LC: The effects of Beta-Aminoproprionitrile after Posterior Penetrating Injury in the Rabbit. *Am J Ophthalmol* 95:97-109, 1983.

Chapter 13

Complications of Radial Keratotomy

Warren D. Cross, MD
Wm. Justus Head, III, MD

COMPLICATIONS OF RADIAL KERATOTOMY

After almost five years of experience with radial keratotomy in the United States and 10 years in the Soviet Union, the rate of complications from this procedure is low.[1-3] The most common complications are overcorrections and undercorrections, while the severe complications such as cataract formation, corneal infection and endophthalmitis are rare. Endothelial cell loss has not proven to be a problem as indicated by several studies which have failed to demonstrate significant or progressive endothelial cell loss. In addition, the already low rate of complications has been decreasing with experience, improved technique, and new instrumentation. The complications experienced or reported include: overcorrections, undercorrections, induced astigmatism, perforation of the cornea, postoperative glare, fluctuation of refraction, reduced night vision, photophobia, reduction of best corrected vision, monocular diplopia or multiple ghost images, need for re-operation, recurrent erosions, inability to wear a contact lens postoperatively, neovascularization of incisions, excessive scarring, epithelial cysts in incisions, exacerbation of epithelial dystrophy, endothelial cell loss, glaucoma, cataract formation, corneal infection, and endophthalmitis. This chapter will discuss the prevention, recognition, and management of these complications.

Operative Complications

Perforations. Perforations of the cornea should be minimized since they may result in loss of the anterior chamber and all associated sequelae (peripheral anterior synechiae, glaucoma, cataract) and can predispose the eye to an endophthalmitis. Cutting through Descemet's membrane could result in increased and/or progressive endothelial cell loss. Theoretically, a perforation also risks development of an epithelial or fibrous downgrowth into the anterior chamber.

Microperforations. Microperforations (Figure 13-1) are defined as self-sealing perforations usually much less than 1 mm in length. The frequency of perforations has been reported to be as high as 35%, but in most studies it has been about 5% to 10%.[1-5] Perforations are more likely to occur in the inferotemporal region (Figure 13-2) of the cornea and are also more likely to occur when redeepening (making peripheral cutdowns). One theory holds that as the operation progresses on a "dry" cornea, surface evaporation and thinning of the cornea by dehydration occurs. As a result the last incisions would be more likely to perforate. This theory has not been proven except in animal studies.[4] Trusting the pachymeter-knife relationship is of utmost importance in avoiding perforations while getting reproducibly deep incisions. This approach requires measuring corneal thickness and setting the blade extension in a tried and proven manner.

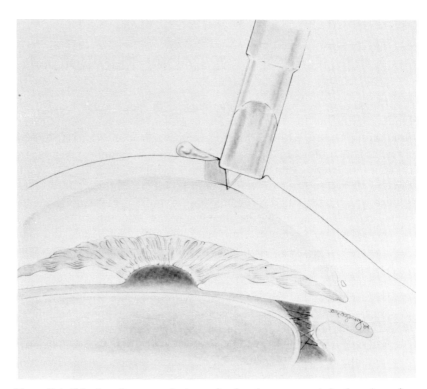

Figure 13-1. Side view of paracentral microperforation. Aqueous percolation from the perforation site usually appears immediately upon entering into the anterior chamber.

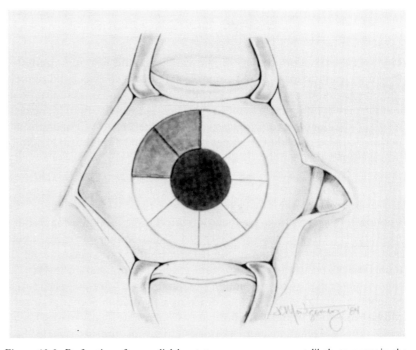

Figure 13-2. Perforations from radial keratotomy surgery are most likely to occur in the inferotemporal quadrant or late in the procedure when the cornea becomes thin and dry. Surgeon's view through operating microscope, left eye.

Measurement in multiple quadrants also may help detect thin regions and allow compensation of the blade setting. The blade should be checked periodically with an atraumatic coin or sliding gauge to verify the setting.

When cutting in the temporal zone, avoid exerting excessive pressure in the midperipheral portion of the incisions. Always use special care when re-deepening incisions; if pressure is exerted when redeepening, the guard of the blade has a tendency to enter the incision, causing perforation (Figure 13-3). The amount of pressure exerted on the knife can influence the incision depth and direction of the incision (Figure 13-4A and B). The amount of counter pressure exerted with the fixation forceps[2] can also affect direction and depth of the incision. Increased intraocular pressure from counter pressure may cause the floor of the incision to bulge upward forcing the blade to cut full thickness. Some micrometer diamond blades now on the market will cut more deeply if not held perfectly perpendicular to the corneal surface. Care must be taken to hold the knife exactly at an angle perpendicular to the corneal surface since in some knife designs "tilting" the knife away from the cutting angle (toward the optical zone) allows the guard to be situated on the curved surface and therefore cut at a greater depth. This phenomenon is more likely to occur with nasal and brow incisions due to anatomic problems with the angle of approach. Hyperextension of the neck and slight rotation of the face (temporal side up) reduce this obstruction (Figure 13-5A and B).

Immediate detection of a perforation is imperative. If the blade enters the anterior chamber, the sudden appearance of a drop of aqueous heralds the point where the blade perforated the cornea. During surgery maintain a dry blade and a corneal surface moistened only slightly with anesthetic solution such as 4% topical lidocaine hydrochloride (Xylocaine) so the knife guard moves easily across the corneal surface. The appearance of the aqueous drop then will be easily detectable. If there is any question about a perforation, aqueous can be detected by drying the suspicious area and then pressing lightly with a dry or "squeezed dry" cellulose sponge. If there is a definite loss of intraocular pressure or a flattening of the anterior

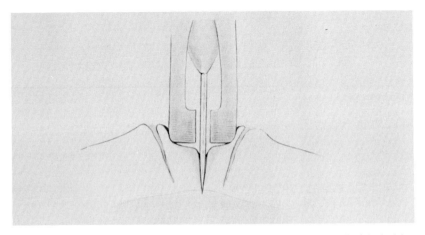

Figure 13-3. Excessive pressure during redeepening tends to spread the wall of the incision apart allowing excessively deep penetration.

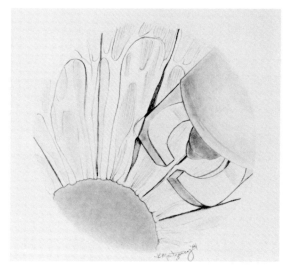

Figure 13-4A. Excessive blade pressure can cause a soft shoulder phenomenon in which the blade guard becomes depressed into the neighboring incisions. This snagging of the footplate can cause blade tilt or misdirection.

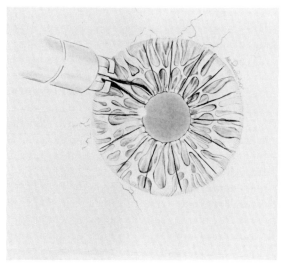

Figure 13-4B. The soft shoulder phenomenon can become severe in a 12- or 16-incision RK such that the misdirected blade will cause extension of the current incision into a neighboring incision. This junction of two incisions can cause irregular astigmatism, lamellar stromal dehiscence and scarring.

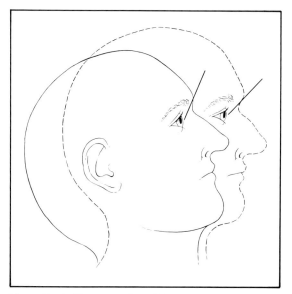

Figure 13-5A. Hyperextension of the neck improves the angle of attack in a patient with a large frontal or brow process.

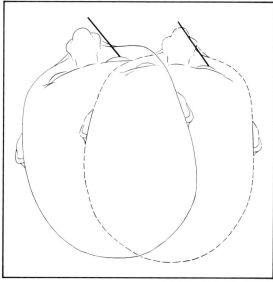

Figure 13-5B. Slight rotation of the face (temporal side up) improves the angle of attack in a patient with a large nose or prominent nasal bridge.

chamber, a macroperforation should be considered. The radial keratotomy surgeon should always be ready to stop his incision the instant a microperforation is detected to avoid extension into a macroperforation.

Microperforations usually are self-sealing as the adjacent corneal stroma swells from contact with the aqueous. As soon as the perforation is sealed (usually in less than one minute), surgery can be continued (but cautiously). Incisions most distant from the perforation should be done next as pressure on the cornea near the perforation can reopen it. If two or three microperforations occur during the case, the blade extension should be reduced by 10 to 20 microns before proceeding. Care should be taken if the blade is re-inserted into a perforated incision as this could result in extension of the perforation. Similarly, an incision with a perforation should not be irrigated as this could introduce foreign material into the anterior chamber. Despite the undesirability of perforations, most of these complications cases can be completed.

When perforation into the anterior chamber has occurred, subconjunctival injection of antibiotics (aminoglycoside and cephalosporin) should be given. Some surgeons advocate subconjunctival steroid injection for iritis which is more likely to occur with perforations, while others do not use a steroid injection for fear of masking an infection should it occur. If there is a question about whether the leak is self-sealed or, in cases of persistent aqueous leaks, a bandage soft contact lens may be used to help maintain the anterior chamber. The bandage soft contact lens should be applied at the time of surgery under aseptic conditions with topical antibiotic drops continued postoperatively. In cases with perforations, the surgeon should examine the patient on the first postoperative day to check for loss of anterior chamber or persistent aqueous leak. Persistent leaks should be treated with suturing if they do not seal with a bandage contact lens in two days. If the perforation is very near the optical axis of the cornea, prudence is indicated to weigh the severity of the persistent leak against the possibility of inducing astigmatism by suturing. A patient with a microperforation, a sutured macroperforation, or a large number of incisions should be instructed to wear a metal shield while asleep to protect the eye. Persistent leakage of a microperforation can be clinically taxing due to the possibility of infection from continued leaking or the suturing causing irritation and astigmatism.

Macroperforations. A macroperforation (Figure 13-6) is a large full-thickness corneal incision which requires suturing to maintain the anterior chamber. With the advent of the diamond micrometer blade, macroperforations became rare, presumably due to the elimination of error associated with hand setting the exposure length of a razor blade fragment into a holder. The increased sharpness of the diamond helps avoid a "plowing" incision of the duller metal blades used in a peripheral to central motion.

Since microperforations can be expected in approximately 5% to 10% of the cases, it is imperative that the radial keratotomy surgeon avoid extension of a self-sealing perforation into one that results in loss of the anterior chamber and requires suturing. This type of perforation also risks damage to the crystalline lens. Once the blade has been adequately inserted to get good depth at the optical zone, the initial outward sweep should be very slow and deliberate, stopping as soon as a perceptible movement of the blade has occurred. If aqueous appears at this point, the blade must be immediately removed to avoid extension of the perforation. If no aqueous appears at this time, the incision can be slowly continued toward the limbus. Care is indicated during the entire incision as thin spots in the corneal peripheral are known to exist.

A macroperforation should be assumed to occur when the anterior chamber depth is decreased (Figure 13-7). This type of perforation should be visible under the operating microscope. Any large perforating corneal incision should be carefully sutured using 10-0 or 11-0 nylon. Single interrupted stitches provide the most control (Figure 13-8). If necessary the anterior chamber can be reformed with balanced salt solution or Healon®. Care should be taken during the repair not to injure the crystalline lens, nor to incarcerate the iris in the incision. Anyone who performs radial keratotomy should be adept at closing a large perforating corneal incision. Subcon-

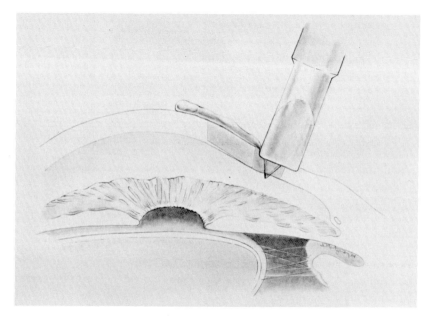

Figure 13-6. Macroperforations are large extensions of unrecognized microperforations which due to excessive aqueous leakage frequently result in chamber shallowing. The risk of chamber collapse, infection, scarring, iris adhesions, and cataract are significantly higher with macroperforations. Macroperforations frequently cause premature cessation of the surgical procedure.

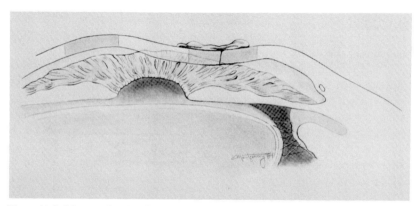

Figure 13-7. Macroperforation frequently causes loss of anterior chamber depth.

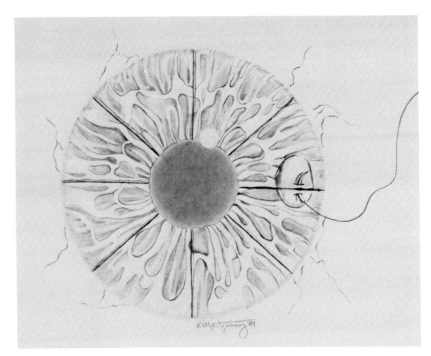

Figure 13-8. Suturing of the macroperforation is frequently the only assured recourse for the surgeon in order to prevent more severe sequellae from developing. The sutures should remain in the cornea for at least three to four weeks. Monofilament 10-0 or 11-0 suture in an interrupted fashion with the knots rotated and buried should provide an asymptomatic solution to the macroperforation dilemma.

junctival antibiotics should be given, and close follow-up is very prudent. Do not remove sutures too soon as this could result in reoccurrence of the leak; one local case required suturing three times due to removal of sutures too soon. One of our cases had a macroperforation on the third incision. Breakdown of the sutured incision with a flat chamber occurred at three weeks postoperatively. Micro-necrotic areas were present around each suture secondary to nylon sensitivity. This was resutured with prolene to which the patient was apparently also sensitive. The wound was finally successfully closed with three 8-0 white silk sutures, which were removed after approximately one month. The patient is now three and one half years postoperative, has had no additional surgery, and has an uncorrected postoperative visual acuity of 20/25+.

Errors of Optical Axis Determination Determination of the optical axis can be accomplished by several techniques. Some surgeons use topical anesthetic to make a corneal mark on the center of the small light reflex with a needle at the slit lamp, while other surgeons have described a technique of marking the corneal light reflex while looking through a direct ophthalmoscope. There are several optical marking devices currently available, including the Osher Centering Device.[2] Most surgeons use the light reflex from the surgical operating microscope for marking the optical axis, assuming the light source is "coaxial." Since in all coaxial microscopes the

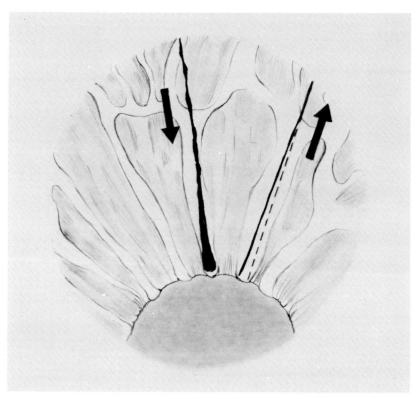

Figure 13-9. Incisions made in the classic peripheral to central mode suffer from three significant problems: (1) due to resistance of the corneal tissue the blade motion is jagged; (2) the central exit site of the blade causes increased scarring due to Bowman's membrane damage; and (3) the risk of entering the optical zone is significantly increased under topical anesthesia or when globe fixation is unstable. The central to peripheral mode may be straight and thin but with current pen shaped blade handles, the exact path of the blade is difficult to match with a reference line. Entry into the optical zone is less likely with the central to peripheral technique.

projected light source is not truly coaxial, the light/reflex relationship for each microscope is different. Therefore, each surgeon must determine from the above techniques and/or the microscope company the light/reflex relationship for each microscope model. In any case this is a unique circumstance in surgery since the decision of the surgeon (marking of the optical center) is totally dependent on the patient looking into the light source and fixating on the light source as instructed. The optical axis should be rechecked two or three times. Some surgeons treat the patient pre-operatively with pilocarpine to decrease photosensitivity while improving the accuracy of the marking. This technique is also facilitated with microscopes having rheostats, or blue/green filters. Remember, the geometric center and optical axis are rarely the same.

Incision Across the Visual Axis. This complication is avoided primarily by making all incisions from the optical zone toward the limbus (Figure 13-9). Control of the eye during the operation is essential to avoid incisions that stray or are oblique. Retrobulbar injection of local anesthetic provides the utmost in control of the eye, but increases surgical morbidity. Fixation is also important: the use of a Thornton fixation ring, Kremer locking forceps, Hofmann forceps, Bores forceps, etc. helps maintain adequate globe fixation and counter rotation while making the incisions. The vacuum fixation ring such as the Barraquer or the Gelender vacuum system has been advocated for maximum control and reproducible depth.[6] Experience with these suction devices is limited in radial keratotomy surgery (Figure 13-10). Control of total patient movement is extremely important; it is best accomplished by good rapport with the patient and sedation of the apprehensive patient.

The best management of this complication is avoidance. Should it occur, explanation to the patient could be very reassuring. The incision should be allowed to heal completely (six months) and vision evaluated before further treatment such as penetrating keratoplasty is undertaken. One reported case resulted in significant overcorrection and induced astigmatism, but corrected vision was 20/25.

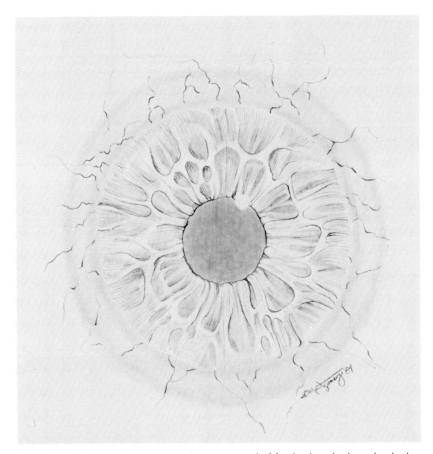

Figure 13-10. Suction fixation devices improve control of fixation but also have drawbacks. They induce peri-limbal chemosis, subconjunctival hemorrhage, increased surgical pain, and they lengthen the procedure time.

Too Many Incisions. The use of a corneal incision marker will help the surgeon account for the number of incisions to be made. Of course, since the number of incisions affects the amount of correction obtained, the radial keratotomy surgeon should count carefully the incisions during surgery. If an extra incision is made, no attempt to make other incisions for symmetry is indicated. Very frequently these patients will do quite well. Asymmetry of the incisions does not as a rule result in unacceptable astigmatism.

Too Few Incisions. Frequently, the result (Figure 13-11) is excellent in cases where the surgery was aborted, possibly due to perforation, or in cases where an incision was inadvertently omitted. If an undercorrection or astigmatism results, appropriate measures should be undertaken. In initial cases the incisions should be 90° to each other as the case is done, because if the case is aborted, less astigmatism will result than if the incisions are 180° from each other.

Wrong Axis on Astigmatism Correction. Avoiding this significant complication involves good understanding of the principles of astigmatism correction and careful preoperative planning for each case. The surgeon should have a very clear idea as to which is the steepest corneal meridian with respect to the axis on the refraction. Radial keratotomy should be done to correct the spherical component of the refraction written in minus cylinder form. The minus cylinder component is then corrected with astigmatism incision(s). The astigmatism correcting incisions are made in the steeper corneal meridian, which is 90° from the axis of the minus cylinder refraction.

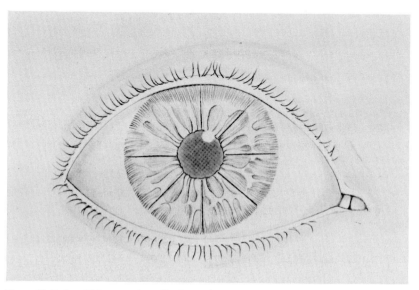

Figure 13-11. Insufficient number of incisions frequently results in no adverse consequences. Missing incisions have less effect if the previous incisions were balanced 90° from each other to avoid astigmatism.

Drawing a sketch of the cornea with proposed incisions in relation to the position of the nose improves the surgeon's orientation. Turning the picture upside down simulates the surgeon's position at the head of the patient. The position of the nose is a good landmark and will prevent confusion when approaching the eye which, from the surgeon's view, is in an upside down position during the operation. At the beginning of the case when marking the optical axis, mark the 90° and 180° axis and the axis of the proposed astigmatism correcting incision(s). This is easily done using a .12 forceps dipped in methylene blue or brilliant green dye with the Mendez astigmatic dial for reference. This method helps to eliminate axis error due to torsion of the eye induced by fixation or retrobulbar block.

If the wrong axis is operated upon, the eye should be allowed to heal for six months before being re-operated. Tapering topical steroids early and the use of timolol maleate (Timoptic) 0.5% twice a day will encourage regression of the effect (see discussion of this in the section on overcorrections).

Incision into the Limbus. Past experience by some surgeons indicates that incision into the limbus could result in a decreased effect. In the Houston study, some patients had increased postoperative pain but no decrease in effect was observed in cases where a few of the incisions entered the limbus inadvertently. Simple visualization and controlled movement of the blade are necessary to prevent excessive extension of the incisions into the limbus. Experience is necessary to judge the extent of the incision as it is created since the blade guard may block direct visualization.

Limbal extension of the incision is managed by carefully irrigating blood from the incision at the end of the case. Cautery should never be used to control bleeding from incisions into the limbal vessels. Cautery scars tend to induce neovascularization of the incision. Avoid fitting contact lenses postoperatively for 12 months to prevent neovascularization of the incisions.

Postoperative Complications

Overcorrection. The rate of overcorrection from radial keratotomy in most hands is 5% to 10%. When an overcorrection occurs, the topical steroid should be tapered early and measures to lower intraocular pressure used. Usually this means timolol maleate, epinephrine, and pilocarpine topically. Oral carbonic anhydrase inhibitors should also be considered. There is no experimental or clinical proof that the pressure in a normotensive eye can be reduced by these drugs or that the mechanism for the decrease in effect is by the reduction of intraocular pressure. However, theoretical considerations of radial keratotomy predict pressure as influencing effect.[1] A reduction in effect can be obtained clinically by using topical miotics and/or timolol maleate early in the postoperative healing phase of radial keratotomy. It is possible that this is simply blunting the diurnal rises in intraocular pressure or that it is suppressing a rise in intraocular pressure associated with topical steroid use. This subject is still open to more intense investigation. The mechanism for the increased regression seen by

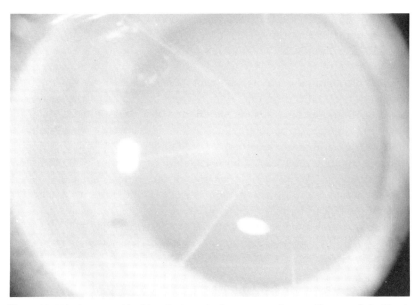

Figure 13-12A. Acute peri-incisional edema in the paracentral zone. (Courtesy L.J. Girard, M.D.)

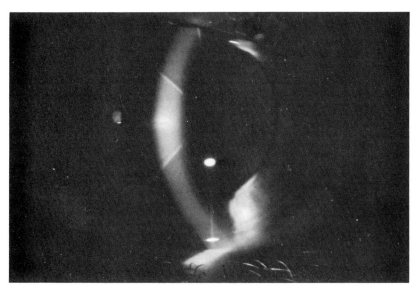

Figure 13-12B. Persistent corneal peri-incisional opacification due to long-term stromal edema. (Courtesy L.J. Girard, M.D.)

stopping postoperative topical steroid also has not been scientifically investigated. In the Houston study, topical steroids were used postoperatively on all patients and the nomogram for optical zone size used is dependent on their effect. The regression with early cessation of steroids may be due to elimination of steroid effect on intraocular pressure or may be related to the suppression of healing produced by steroids.

In patients 20 to 30 years old 1 diopter to 2 diopters of persistent hyperopia will usually regress in three to four months without intervention.

In older patients the regression is not spontaneous but can be encouraged by tapering steroids early and using ocular hypotensive agents. For treatment of overcorrections Schachar[3] has advocated reopening incisions after an adequate postoperative healing period and allowing them to heal again under the effect of ocular hypotensive agents. The authors have no personal experience with this technique.

Increased hydration of the cornea has been implicated in pathogenesis of overcorrections.[3] In the immediate postoperative period there is swelling of the cornea around the incisions with resultant overcorrection (Figures 13-12A and B). As healing of the epithelium occurs with re-establishment of a barrier to fluid entrance, corneal hydration decreases and the excessive effect of the incisions diminishes. In some cases there may be a prolonged delay in re-establishment of epithelial integrity with persistent overcorrection in what is theorized to be a "leaking epithelium syndrome." This can occur in patients who initially have a good correction and return later having developed an overcorrection. Frequently the problem may only affect some incisions giving the increased correction only along this axis. The refraction will usually reflect good correction in one axis and the overcorrection 90° away, e.g. +3.00-3.00 × 45. This is sometimes seen with astigmatism-correcting cross-hatch or T-incisions. Delayed healing or prolonged epithelial leakage can result in large overcorrection of the cylinder. Sometimes fluorescein can be seen to rapidly penetrate deep into the incision demonstrating the lack of healing even several months postoperatively. It is very important to recognize this problem and avoid re-operation until a prolonged recovery is allowed. Use of 5% sodium chloride drops and ointment is recommended. The mechanism of action theorized is reduction of the abnormal corneal hydration. Other measures for dealing with overcorrections should also be followed. Topical steroids should be avoided in patients demonstrating this poor healing response.

Overcorrections can occur in patients who have an elevated intraocular pressure or in patients who develop an elevated pressure in response to topical steroid treatment. A thicker cornea is also associated with increased correction. Overcorrection may be associated with delayed healing of the incisions, which is especially true of astigmatism incisions. Permanent overcorrection is more common in patients over 40 and the older patient is unable to compensate for a small hyperopia by accommodation. On the other hand, small overcorrections less than 1 diopter in the young patient usually provide good vision.

The authors try to avoid large overcorrections to the point of erring on the undercorrection side since the lifelong myope often has trouble adapting to hyperopia. The explanation for this involves control of accommodation and the accommodation-convergence system. A person who has always been myopic has not learned to maintain a tonic accommodation to compensate for hyperopia and so experiences trouble focusing even though he can with 20/20 acuity. Myopes have learned to converge without accommodation when not wearing correction; the need to accommodate while converging as occurs in hyperopia is opposite to the accustomed situation. The patient with small residual myopia post-radial keratotomy usually has a vision better than the refraction would suggest. A residual −0.75 diopter post-RK may have 20/25 vision uncorrected. This is explained by the production of an aspherical corneal curvature post-RK in which a beneficial effect on visual acuity is produced.[1]

Progressive Hyperopia. Elevated intraocular pressure postoperatively either due to steroid response or from development of open angle glaucoma can cause hyperopia in a patient who initially has a good response to radial keratotomy. One case reported in Houston had a preoperative pressure of 22 mm Hg OD and 28 mm Hg OS, preoperative refraction was −4.50 OD and −4.75 OS. Five weeks after surgery his refraction was −1.25 OD and plano-0.50×180 OS. Over the next two years his pressure was repeatedly elevated and required initiation of pilocarpine, timolol maleate, dipivefrin and finally, acetazolamide for control. Intraocular pressure ranged from 17 to 28 OD and 19 to 34 OS. After two years his refraction was +1.50-1.00×45 OD and +4.25-1.25×45 OS. This intraocular pressure rise caused an increase of approximately 0.2 diopters for each 1 mm Hg rise.

Undercorrection. The rate of significant undercorrection in most experienced surgeons' series is about 10%. Unexpected significant undercorrections are primarily associated with shallow incisions which can be the result of inaccurate pachymetry, poor technique, improper blade setting, or a dull blade. It is believed that the protein build-up or chipping against metal depth gauges with diamond blades is the cause of their "dulling." Appropriate frequent cleaning is necessary to keep a diamond blade free of protein build-up. Patients with a low intraocular pressure may experience an undercorrection especially if intraocular pressure is less than eight to 10 mm Hg. Young females and patients with thin corneas also seem to be prone to undercorrection. Small undercorrections do not necessarily result in unhappy patients as the vision is usually better than the residual myopia would suggest. It is thought that even with undercorrection radial keratotomy produces an optically beneficial change in the cornea.[1] Patients do not always adapt well to being changed from myopes to low hyperopes so erring on the side of undercorrection is wise.

Undercorrection, especially in the nondominant eye in the early presbyopia patient is probably the best result possible. Most surgeons attempt to leave these people with −.75 diopter to 1.25 diopters if possible. If the patient is unable to tolerate the undercorrection and a good result is obtained in the dominant eye, the surgeon may consider adjustment after nine to 12 months.

The most common cause of undercorrection or overcorrection is the incorrect choice of surgical treatment for the patient's refraction. The authors use from four radial incisions to a maximum of 16 incisions and vary the optical zone from 3.0 mm to 5.0 mm for radial keratotomy and for Ruiz procedures. A nomogram is included (Chapter 5) for assistance, indicating many clinical parameters influencing the surgical design. The potential radial keratotomy surgeon should remember that one can always add additional incisions if needed but erasing too many or enlarging a too small an optical zone cannot be done! This should always be explained to every patient preoperatively and that a second procedure or "adjustment" may be needed in 5% to 10% of cases. Undercorrection is obviously much more likely to occur in the 18 to 20 year old age group. Corrections greater than

−5.00 to −5.50 are very difficult to attain in this age group and high myopia should be treated with myopic keratomileusis or epikeratophakia.

Intraocular pressure is a significant predictive factor in all ages, but especially in the young patient. Any patient with tonometry of 8 to 10 mm Hg or less should be informed that the surgical prognosis for obtaining a large correction is poor. Eyes with tonometry of 8 to 10 mm receive very little correction (especially in younger patients) and although they initially look good, they eventually regress severely almost without exception. Of the over 4,000 cases in the Houston Study there are seven such patients with postoperative refractions almost identical with preoperative refraction. The most notable case was that of a 19-year-old white male with a refraction of −5.50 sphere OD and −5.25 OS. His intraocular pressure by applanation was 10 mm Hg. Three years ago a 3.0 optical zone 16 incision radial keratotomy was done with a diamond blade set at 95% depth. The surgery was repeated with peripheral redeepening one year postoperatively. Three years postoperatively the stable refraction was −4.50-0.50×180 OD and −5.00 OS. With his informed consent, treatment with oral steroids, sub-Tenons steroids, and steroid drops were used to no avail. In the Houston Study a patient with a low intraocular pressure preoperatively has never been a steroid responder.

Assuming the correct surgical design is chosen, the next most common cause of undercorrection is incorrect hand, knife, eye, and head position resulting in shallow incisions. Current understanding indicates that the depth of the incisions near the optical zone is most critical. The incisions must be absolutely perpendicular both vertically to the optical axis as well as to the surface of the cornea. Incisions not perpendicular at the optical zone produce the effect of a larger optical zone and therefore less correction. Incisions oblique to the corneal surface (tilted right or left) are too shallow, causing reduced surgical effect, and they increase glare due to diffraction. An improved angle of attack decreases the awkwardness of hand and instrument placement in some quadrants. Hyperextension of the head (by placing a pillow under the shoulder) tilts the brow and bridge of the nose away from the surgeon's hand allowing greater access to the eye. Turning the face to the opposite side and abducting the operative eye also improves exposure.

It would be prudent for the beginning radial keratotomy surgeon to initiate radial keratotomies at well-spaced intervals so that his surgical technique and results can be evaluated. Every incision should be studied at the slit lamp postoperatively (especially at the insertion) as to depth, vertical relationship to optical axis, and perpendicularity to the cornea. The use of a retinal drawing sheet to sketch the incisions of each case of the first 50 cases is advisable to allow the surgeon to see the pattern of his surgical errors. Most technical errors involve incisions made over the brow and/or bridge of the nose (i.e. shallow, wrong angle, not perpendicular, etc.). Look at every incision, then try to correct poor technique on the subsequent cases. Failure to learn from each case gives the novice refractive surgeon cases which may look good initially, but as the healing occurs, undercorrections, regular and/or irregular astigmatism may develop six months to two years later with the surgeon having little insight into the etiology. Surgeons having videotape capabilities should find critical review of recorded surgical technique helpful to avoid future technical errors.

For significant undercorrections additional correction may be obtained with repeat surgery. The surgeon should wait three to four months before re-operating a routine eight-incision radial keratotomy to allow sufficient healing of the incisions so that regression and fluctuation have stabilized. For 12- and 16-incision radial keratotomy repeat surgery should wait six months to one year. For patients with astigmatism-correcting incisions it is necessary to wait six months to a year for stabilization. A re-operation should be done if the patient desires it and the surgeon feels he can get additional correction. If the uncorrected vision is 20/40 or better the indication for re-operation is questionable. Examine the patient at the slit lamp: look for shallow incisions and measure the optical zone in several axes using the slit beam. If there is an opportunity to make a smaller optical zone and/or deeper incisions, additional correction can be obtained. If there is a 3.0 mm optical zone (without some incisions falling short) with 16 deep incisions, the chance for additional correction is nil. Peripheral redeepening can get 5% additional correction but care must be taken in cutting into old incisions. There may be thin spots resulting in perforation, excessive scarring, and cyst formation. The authors avoid re-operating more than once due to the high risk of irregular astigmatism and cicatrization.

The surgical treatment of undercorrection is a very difficult problem because the amount of correction obtained in a previously operated eye is considerably less than that obtained in a non-operated eye provided the original surgery was done at 90% depth with good insertion technique at the optical zone. In these cases a minimum of four to six incisions is necessary to effect any significant spherical changes. Some surgeons prefer peripheral redeepening and describe good results; others simply add four to eight new incisions. In cases where the incisions were shallow, the surgeon has a greater risk of overcorrection if he does the second procedure technically well at the 90% depth, especially in patients over 35 years old. It may be advisable for the novice surgeon to consult with an experienced surgeon in determining the parameters (optical zone, number of incisions, incision pattern) of a re-operation.

Determining the optical axis in a re-operation is occasionally a major problem for the RK surgeon since it may not match the original optical axis as marked. Make certain the original optical zone is identified before doing a re-operation. Every attempt should be made to avoid making incisions which encroach into the optical zone. This is or can be one of the most difficult decisions in refractive surgery and, at this time, no clear answer seems to exist. Generally, if the residual refractive error is spherical, the initial optical axis can be used. If the residual refraction is astigmatic and incisions all look technically correct, the surgeon should suspect misalignment of the original optical axis. If initial misalignment has occurred, an attempt is made to make the new axis halfway between the original axis and the "new apparent axis," taking care to preserve as much of the non-incised central corneal area as possible. After nine to 12 months, residual astigmatism can generally be treated surgically with proper cross-hatch incisions.

How to Avoid Shallow Incisions. Good technique involves a firm

hand in every incision. It should also be observed that continual pressure on the globe decreases intraocular pressure such that the cornea is not pressed against the blade as firmly in cases taking an extensive amount of time and/ or a large number of incisions. The later incisions may be shallower due to less pressure so that, depending on their location, this may led to undercorrection and/or astigmatism. Some radial keratotomy surgeons use 3 to 5 cc retrobulbar (xylocaine/Marcaine) or extraconal injection to proptose the eyes of these cases. Some feel that a Thornton scleral ring (which produces external scleral pressure) allows the surgeon to increase the intraocular pressure for the incision and circumvents this problem. Several suction rings are available to prevent this problem. There is no doubt that the eye is made firm by using these suction devices but if perforation occurs, the inherent risks of chamber collapse appear to be much greater. They are, however, very effective at giving a firm cornea to incise under controlled uncomplicated circumstances. The surgeon should also be aware of the increased risks of microperforation, surgical pain, conjunctival chemosis, subconjunctival hemorrhage and increased operative time with these devices.

Anisometropia. Some patients who have very high refractive errors and are treated with a radial keratotomy in one eye can have anisometropia as an interesting complication. One Houston patient had a refractive error of −9.00 OU and was corrected to 20/30 in one eye. The patient had problems from glare as a small optical zone had been used. As a result he refused surgery on the other eye and now has a problem with anisometropia. Another patient had only one eye operated upon due to poor result, having gone from a −6.00 to a +3.00. He now has a problem with anisometropia, being −6.00 in the unoperated eye, and is intolerant to contact lens wear. Conversely one patient who is a physician had only one eye done and went from −13.00 to −3.00. He is awaiting a myopic keratomileusis in the other eye but has no complaints from his anisometropia.

Residual and Induced Astigmatism. Induced astigmatism up to 1.00 diopter following radial keratotomy is not uncommon and usually is compatible with excellent uncorrected vision. The spherical equivalent in most cases is near plano. However, there is an occasional patient who may have a large astigmatism postoperatively. This astigmatism is more common when trying to correct extreme amounts of myopia with 16 incisions and redeepening. Perforations are sometimes associated with induced astigmatism but this is not always the case. Perforations usually do not seem to induce astigmatism but, in cases with multiple perforations, astigmatism is sometimes seen. Overcorrection from astigmatism correction incisions is another source of postoperative astigmatism. If the surgery for the spherical component was correct, then the patient becomes a compound hyperope with the axis 90° away from the original axis. In this case the patient may respond to tapering steroids early and lowering intraocular pressure. The "leaking epithelium syndrome" with stromal edema can also result in a transient induced astigmatism.

Residual astigmatism is the result of not surgically correcting the astigmatism, inadequately correcting the astigmatism by poor techniques, choosing the incorrect method for the degree of cylinder (based on refraction, age, and intraocular pressure), or the nonrecognition of lenticular astigmatism. For surgeons performing their first 50 to 100 cases in patients with less than 1.00 to 1.25 cylinder preoperatively, perhaps no attempt to correct the astigmatism should be made. This is because the inexperienced surgeon may induce an unpredictable amount of cylinder at an unknown axis.

Initial attempts to correct astigmatism should be made in patients with low degrees of astigmatism (-0.75 to -2.00). This range can be managed by "cross-hatch" incisions or "T-cuts." Much of the past criticism of this technique's unpredictable results was due to the incisions being about one-third to one-half the distance along the length of the radial incision. Poor results occurred in patients with large corneas (13.0 to 14.5 mm) since the incisions were greater distances from the optical zone/optical center. By always doing cross-hatch or T-cut incisions with a 6 mm to 7 mm optical zone and a 4 mm length, the radial keratotomy surgeon's result will be more predictable and quantifiable. Care should be taken to misalign slightly the cross-hatch incisions especially at the three and nine o'clock positions. In older patients with drooping lower lids, the six o'clock incision will frequently heal slowly. Perfect alignment of incisions frequently causes the corneal "tips" to melt and the wound will heal more slowly due to "fish-mouthing." Two cross-hatch incisions will correct greater amounts of cylinder but also increase the amount of scarring. If clinically indicated, cross-hatch incisions closer to the optical axis will give more correction of astigmatism but may also increase the chances for glare, "starburst," monocular diplopia or triplopia, e.g., a 37-year-old white male with a preoperative refraction of plano -5.50×180 had a 3.0 mm optical zone radial keratotomy with a cross-hatch at the 3.5 mm optical zone. This patient now has a refraction of $+0.25$-0.50×180 after three and one half years. The patient's visual acuity is 20/25+ without any glare or complaints. These incisions, however, were so close to the optical axis that the eye required daily artificial tears with lubricant ointment and patching at bedtime for several months to aid healing. However, currently, the Ruiz procedure would be the surgeon's first choice, although its glare and distortion due to the central transverse portions of the trapezoid incision are only now beginning to be documented.

In designing the astigmatism procedure, be certain to divide the operation in three parts:

1. Determine the optical zone and the number of incisions for the myopic (spherical) component;
2. Determine what astigmatism correction is necessary; and
3. Determine if correction of the cylinder will influence the spherical component 90° away.

Do not design the surgery based on the spherical equivalent. The refraction -1.25 -4.50×180 has a spherical equivalent of -3.50. If a radial keratotomy is done for -3.50, the patient will have a postoperative result which is actually a compound hyperopia with the axis reversed 90°. This result is very difficult to adjust. The surgeon should think of the refraction in two parts and if confused, draw an optical cross.

Better yet, he should consult with an experienced refractive surgeon adept at planning astigmatic surgery.

The Ruiz procedure works effectively for 2.50 diopters to 8.00 diopters of cylinder correction depending on age, intraocular pressure, spherical refraction, etc. In consideration of inducing myopia, note that the longer the transverse incisions (length of cross-hatch, T-cuts, width of Ruiz "tops") the more the sphere is changed 90° away. This coupling phenomenon can be useful in treating compound hyperopes either primarily or to adjust postoperative problems. A 4.5 mm to 5.0 mm wide cross-hatch or Ruiz procedure allows the surgeon to adjust some cases of compound hyperopia mentioned above. For example, a primary compound hyperope 32 years old with +4.25-7.50×180 OD and +4.00-7.50×180 OS was done with a Ruiz incision of 4.5 mm transverse length. Postoperatively, his refraction was +3.50 sphere OD and +3.75-.75×180 OS at one year. He is able to wear Permalens and is very pleased.

The failure to identify axial or lenticular astigmatism may give the radial keratotomy surgeon a spherical cornea with residual cylinder. Always check the preoperative refraction and keratometry readings for those special patients. These lenticular cylinder patients may be operated upon to correct the "refraction" and not the cornea. The results generally have been acceptable in the Houston study, but extreme caution should be taken and results are less predictable because the surgery is not always in the steepest corneal meridian.

The best treatment of postoperative residual astigmatism is "tincture of time." If re-operation is necessary and it is obvious from the first postoperative examination, make do the adjustment when the second eye is done, thus saving additional hospital costs. If you have your own surgical unit, it is best to wait. Also, the longer the wait (eight to 12 months) the less likely the need to adjust. A large percentage (probably 50%) of the patients seen at four to eights months who appear to need an adjustment return at one year for probable adjustments and do not need, require, or wish to have adjustments. Most radial keratotomy surgeons do not believe in orthokeratology but an argument can be made for the part-time fitting of an oxygen permeable lens as a "splint." With the proper curvature on the healing eye with numerous symmetrically placed incisions the cornea may heal symmetrically (especially in young patients with tight lids). In the Houston study, this modified form of orthokeratology has worked in two-thirds of 20 patients and may be worth the try for four to six months. The use of the contact lens splint appeared to be helpful but the series is too small (20) to make any significant judgment. In certain rare patients, the correction of astigmatism simply does not occur regardless of surgical design. Certain authors feel these patients have an oval shaped annulus or limbus, or may be early undiagnosed keratoconus patients. These are about 5% or less of astigmatism patients.

Detail-oriented patients (engineers, architects, hunters, policemen) will complain much more, often vociferously, if the cylinder is in the dominant eye than if it is in the non-dominant eye. If the residual cylinder is in the non-dominant eye and they do not complain, leave the cylinder alone.

If there is a postoperative myopic astigmatism, re-operation can reduce it. In cases of hyperopic astigmatism and compound astigmatism, a re-operation may result in hyperopia. In cases of hyperopic or compound astigmatism, measures to promote regression of effect should be used. In this way a myopic astigmatism may result which is amenable to surgical intervention. For large cylinder and in compound or hyperopic astigmatism, a Ruiz procedure may result in less hyperopia. Careful consideration should be made before operating on a compound hyperope with a refraction having the conoid of Sturm straddling the retina and an uncorrected vision of 20/25 to 20/40. If the RK surgeon is unsuccessful, the patient will be a pure hyperope which may be a much worse result postoperatively.

Photosensitivity, Starburst, Fluctuation of Vision. Most patients experience these symptoms of distortion which can be quite extreme in the immediate postoperative period. These symptoms, however, invariably improve with time and only occasionally persist longer than six months. Persistent cases are usually associated with smaller optical zone sizes (especially smaller than 3.0 mm), 12 or 16 incisions and with redeepening. Shallow incisions seem to be associated with more fluctuation of vision, as has been reported.[2]

The surgeon can minimize these symptoms when possible by never using an optical zone smaller than 3.0 mm, and by using myopic keratomileusis or epikeratophakia for the large amounts of myopia. The use of a diamond knife in the central to peripheral cutting direction reduces paracentral scarring and tissue trauma. Postoperative steroids topically also reduce scarring with its attendant problems. Symptomatic morning blur due to corneal edema can be clinically reduced by 5% sodium chloride drops during the day and ointment at bedtime.

Glare. Glare after radial keratotomy is rarely greater than that with a contact lens and resolves in most cases after four to eight months. In 5% of patients symptomatic glare may persist for up to one year. Fortunately, as sharper knives have become available and techniques have improved, the problem of glare has been reduced. The careful irrigation of blood, epithelial cells, talc, etc. immediately after surgery helps to assure faint postoperative incisions. If glare is a persistent complaint, it is treated with a drop of 1% topical steroid daily for two to six weeks. In most patients, this greatly decreases the complaint.

With certain patients such as pilots, policemen, firemen, truck drivers, etc. selection of the largest optical zone possible may be very important in reducing symptoms of glare and starburst. If the refractive surgeon determines that such a need exists, a minimum 3.5 mm optical zone should be maintained if possible. A definite relationship exists between optical zone and the number of incisions and/or peripheral redeepening.

$$3.0/8 = 3.5/12$$
$$3.0/12 = 3.5/16$$

After consideration, the surgeon may elect to use a 3.5 mm optical zone with 12 incisions for a case where a 3.0 optical zone with eight incisions would be expected to produce full correction. The surgeon also could choose a 3.5 mm optical zone with peripheral redeepening of the incisions at the 5 mm zone (two zones) to accomplish the same effect. This may be preferable since it leaves more cornea for further incisions if adjustments are necessary. In the Houston study, most patients preferred the eye with the 3.5 mm optical zone over the eye with the 3.0 mm optical zone (they were not told the difference between the two eyes). The surgeon's decision to make additional incisions in the cornea must consider the patient's specific visual requirements, expectations and the radial keratotomy surgeon's philosophy.

Diminished Night Vision.
Diminished night vision is associated with small residual myopia that increases at night due to dilation of the pupil. Pupillary dilation brings into effect the steeper peripheral aspheric cornea, loss of the pinhole effect of the small pupil, and the shift of the light spectrum to favor the blue end (chromatic aberration). Adequate correction or even a small overcorrection will minimize this problem, but some patients may be required to wear corrective lenses to see clearly at night. Refraction for these glasses should be done in a very dark refraction lane without cycloplegia.

Monocular Diplopia and Multiple Ghost Images.
Monocular diplopia and "ghost" images occur occasionally and are seen in patients who have had radial keratotomy with a small optical zone, many incisions, with astigmatism-correcting T-incisions and, especially, with the Ruiz procedure. It is felt that this phenomenon results from placing the incisions too close to the optical axis, especially if the optical axis is not well centered. In all but very few patients these symptoms are temporary and decrease with time as do other visual symptoms like glare, starburst, and fluctuation.

Distortion of Image Perception.
The change in the optical image size, compared to that provided by glasses, is certainly one of the great benefits of refractive surgery. The refractive surgeon must be sensitive to other alterations, especially irregular alterations of perception. This distortion is not an uncommon complaint or observation particularly if the patient is carefully questioned. Patients with previously high myopia may be able postoperatively to "read" the Snellen chart very well. However, many patients have vague complaints about their vision such as difficulty seeing at night, altered depth perception, decreased judgment of distance, or tilting of objects. Decreased night vision seems to be due to a combination of induced glare from multiple incisions and the loss of pinhole effect at night. The 3 mm central area is refractively plano, but past the paracentral region it progresses in an aspheric manner to -1.00, -2.00, -3.00, -4.00, -5.00, -6.00, etc. to the original preoperative refraction of the eye at the limbus. The complaint and observations of the patients are very similar to those seen years ago when the first soft contact lenses were fit which had a very small optically correct central optical zone.

Fitting glasses for a patient with this night vision complaint must be done in a room absolutely dark except for projection chart since this is when the patient has the greatest complaint. Most of these patients are young and in the darkness have pupils which dilate largely (5 mm to 8 mm).

Occasionally, the use of pilocarpine before driving at night is also useful to some of these patients. Patients with small pupillary apertures are much less bothered at night.

Patients with previously high amounts of steep vertical cylinder (3 diopters to to 8 diopters "with the rule") may complain of monocular diplopia or triplopia after surgery. The patient will hold the hands horizontally top and bottom and describe seeing clearly only centrally, better "between the hands," or if they "squint." They complain that they see "double," "triple images," "vision is narrowed," "things tilt away at the top and bottom" etc. Fortunately, as the cornea heals and the brain makes the mental adjustment to the new situation, these complaints disappear by six to 18 months. This may be part of the "normalization of refraction" some authors describe.

Large astigmatic corrections using the Ruiz technique produce increased distortion and complaints. These corneas tend to heal more slowly and the patient must be reassured. Use of 5% NaCl ophthalmic ointment after the cornea is completely re-epithelialized may help shorten the period of the patient's distortion and complaints. Ruiz technique patients are further bothered because frequently the perception 90° away has been changed (especially in the compound hyperopic astigmatic patients).

Poor Healing of Astigmatism Incisions. Care must be taken when performing astigmatism-correcting incisions as the nature of the incision makes them tend to heal poorly (Figures 13-13A and B). These incisions tend to be kept open by collagen fiber separation, lid action, and trauma such as eye rubbing (Figures 13-14A and B). When making a T-incision the tangential part should be done in two steps cutting towards the radial incision and not meeting precisely so that there is a small offset. This will make a better healing incision. Also, the tangential incision should not cross more than one incision since isolating a portion of the cornea away from the limbus will result in difficulty of epithelial healing (Figures 13-15 and 13-16). Care should be taken with the Ruiz type incisions to connect only the central tangential incision with the radial incision; otherwise this could isolate an area of cornea with resultant poor epithelial healing (Figures 13-17 to 13-19) or a stromal "cheese board" effect (Figure 13-20). The Houston study includes three patients who had a Ruiz procedure and subsequently developed elevation of the trapezoid section after rubbing the eye. Two of these required a bandage contact lens to heal, one required prolonged patching to heal. A third patient developed asymptomatic scarring of the stroma in the central half of the trapezoid without any loss of vision.

Reduced Best Corrected Vision. Reduced corrected vision has been an unusual problem in reported experience. Eccentricity of the optical zone producing distortion is the usual cause. Rarely, uneven healing results in an irregular astigmatism with reduced acuity. Cuts across the visual axis or development of a media opacity are other possible causes of visual loss. In patients with the development of a large postoperative astigmatism, especially compound hyperopic astigmatism, there may be a

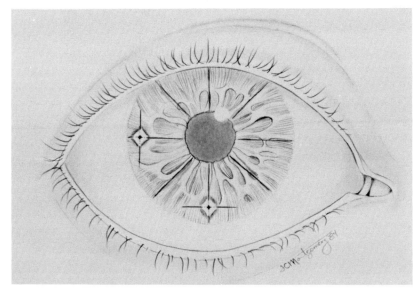

Figure 13-13A. T-cuts joining at the radial incision frequently cause a "fish-mouth" phenomenon with stromal pouting, tip melting, and a diamond-shaped scar.

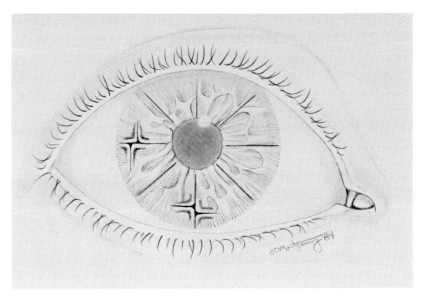

Figure 13-13B. Step T-cut incisions can also cause an offset swastika-shaped incision due to stromal melting and poor wound healing.

decrease in best corrected vision due to distortion. If the patient has severe glare there may be a significant loss of contrast sensitivity. Macular degeneration and retinal hemorrhage from a Fuch's spot after radial keratotomy were felt to be coincidental occurrences. In the Houston study there was one 60-year-old white female who developed a macular hole 6 months after an uncomplicated radial keratotomy. Corneal opacification from a corneal dystrophy or after a corneal ulcer are also known to have caused decreased final visual acuity.

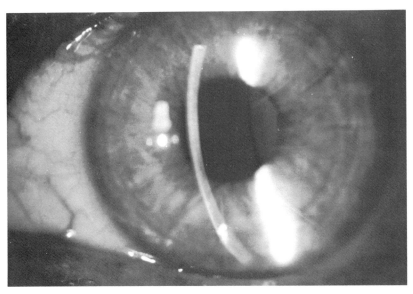

Figure 13-14A. T-cut scarring is due to the transverse release of tension with consequent wound gape and fibrous ingrowth.

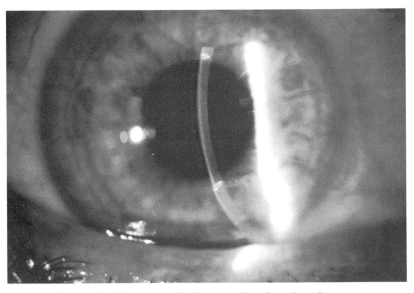

Figure 13-14B. Ruiz incision scarring is due to tension releas along the upper transverse portion of the trapezoid. Frequently this scarring can cause permanent glare and image distortion.

Postoperative Inflammation. Intraocular inflammation is a rare sequela to radial keratotomy. Very infrequently the patient will have a mild anterior chamber reaction a few days postoperatively. One case reported to the Gulf Coast Refractive Keratoplasty Society had both eyes operated one week apart. Three days after surgery the second eye developed a severe iritis which then involved the other eye two days later. The marked fibrinoid anterior chamber reaction required oral and topical steroids for

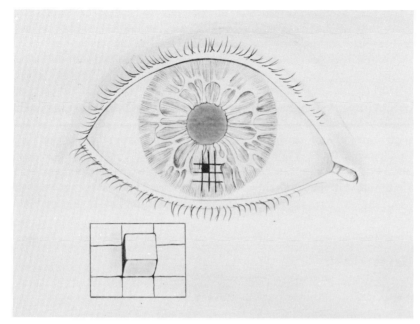

Figure 13-15. Connection of neighboring radial incision with more than one tangential incision results in the "cheese board" effect with lamellar stromal dehiscence. Cross-hatch, T-cut, Ruiz, and mutiple TR cuts all can cause this phenomenon. Perforation with this phenomenon is extremely difficult to close by primary suture repair.

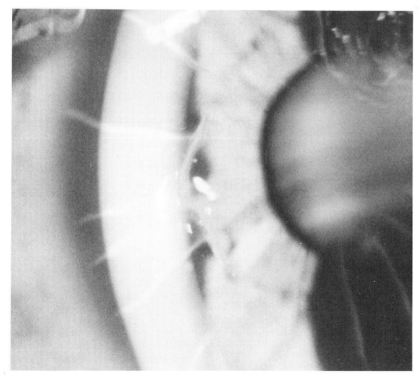

Figure 13-16. Clinical photo of lamellar stromal dehiscence and wound gape from the "cheese board" effect in a T-cut incision which crossed three radial lines. (Courtesy L.J. Girard, M.D.)

treatment. The reaction was severe enough to elevate the intraocular pressure to 48 mm Hg, producing corneal edema. Another reported case developed a sterile hypopyon three days after radial keratotomy which responded well to treatment with topical and locally injected corticosteroids.

Infections: Corneal Ulcer and Endophthalmitis. Infections are very rare following radial keratotomy surgery. Estimates of the frequency are difficult to obtain but appear to be similar to the reported rates for cataract surgery. There have been four cases of endophthalmitis postradial keratotomy reported to the authors' knowledge. One of these cases was reported in the ophthalmic literature (Figure 13-21).[7] Three more cases

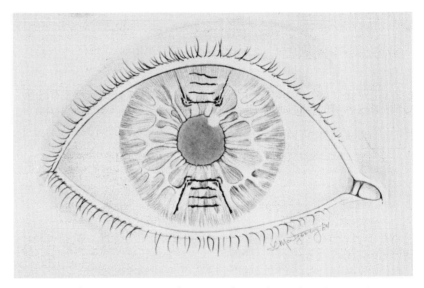

Figure 13-17. Ruiz incision corners frequently elevate along a fault line resulting in poor epithelial healing at the corner of th trapezoid.

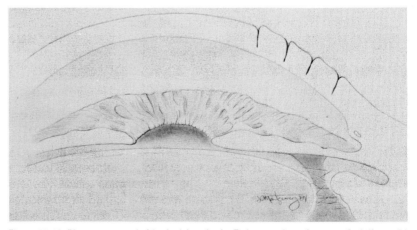

Figure 13-18. Transverse stepladder incisions in the Ruiz procedure also cause fault lines with stromal exposure, tension release, gaping, poor epithelial healing, and resultant scarring.

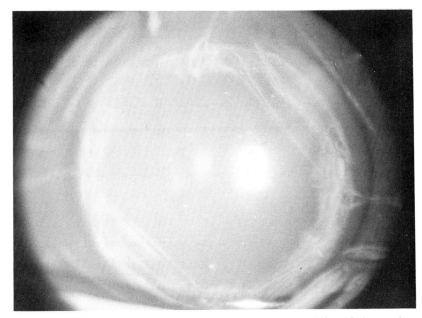

Figure 13-19. Clinical photograph of severe scarring from combined RK and Ruiz procedure with poor technique and a small optical zone. (Courtesy L.J. Girard, M.D.)

have been reported at meetings of the Gulf Coast Refractive Keratoplasty Society. Among the surgeons of this group there have been approximately 25,000 procedures done, making the rate of endophthalmitis to be about 1:8,300. In one of these cases there was placement of a bandage contact lens in the office two to three days postoperatively to control a persistent leak from perforation. The endophthalmitis was treated successfully but the patient subsequently developed a cataract which was removed 18 months after refractive surgery. The authors feel that, because of this, the bandage contact lens, if used, should be placed at the time of surgery under aseptic conditions. One case of endophthalmitis occurred three weeks after surgery when the cornea was inadvertently scratched with a mascara brush. Since a microperforation had occurred during the operation, a tract existed allowing rapid progression to intraocular involvement. The organism isolated was *Pseudomonas*. After hospital treatment final vision was 20/30 best corrected.

There has been one reported case of bacterial corneal ulcer[7] after radial keratotomy in the literature. There have been seven cases of bacterial corneal ulcers reported in Houston out of 25,000 radial keratotomies, giving a rate of about 1:3,500. Four were due to *Pseudomonas* infection and two were *Staphylococcus aureus*. Two of these cases occurred as a bilateral infection with *Pseudomonas* two months after surgery. One case occurred six months and another two years after RK. One of the cases was reported to occur six weeks postoperatively when a cross-hatch incision was opened by rubbing the eye.

Due to the real risk of developing a vision-threatening infection the authors advise performing radial keratotomy surgery in a controlled aseptic operating room environment, utilizing careful antiseptic preparation and

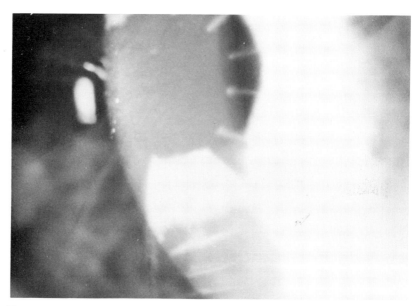

Figure 13-20. Severe paracentral scarring from a "cheese board" effect with stromal dehiscence in a Ruiz/RK combined procedure. (Courtesy L.J. Girard, M.D.)

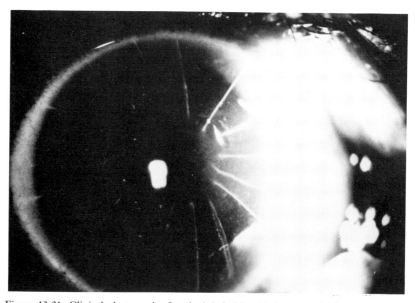

Figure 13-21. Clinical photograph of endophthalmitis with hypopyon 72 hours post-radial keratotomy. (Courtesy H. Gelender, M.D.)

draping procedures. The radial keratotomy procedure has the potential to unexpectedly or unknowingly become an intraocular procedure. Should a corneal ulcer or endophthalmitis be encountered, appropriate aggressive treatment should be immediately instituted.

Rupture of the Globe. The possibility of radial keratotomy predisposing to rupture of the globe by minor trauma has been of major concern to surgeons. In animal studies, weakening of the globe immediately postoperatively has been shown.[8] Another study[9] has shown greater susceptibility to rupture over a 90 day period postoperatively and increased risk of rupture in corneas with microperforations. John[10] has reported a case of severe blunt trauma with a 75% hyphema in a human eye six months post-radial keratotomy without rupture of the globe. In the Houston study there was a patient who parachute-jumped one week after having radial keratotomy with 16 incisions and 3.0 mm optical zone without having any problems. The study also included a similar patient who was struck in the operated eye by a racquetball one week postoperatively and experienced severe pain with iritis; the cornea was intact. One eye was lost following a 60 mph automobile accident into a concrete abutment. The patient was in intensive care for six weeks with multiple facial fractures, severe neurologic injuries, and multiple fractures. Numerous patients have had accidental blows to their eyes (by children, spouses, pets, etc.) without ruptures of the cornea.

Cataract. There has been one reported case[11] of a cataract developing two to three months after radial keratotomy which was uneventful other than a microperforation (Figures 13-22 and 13-23). The etiology of this cataract was unclear as no damage to the lens was apparent from the surgery. Another cataract was reported to have developed following a perforation during a re-deepening procedure.[12] One cataract was reported[7] to have developed in an eye which had had an endophthalmitis after radial keratotomy 18 months prior.

Glaucoma. This complication has not been reported following radial keratotomy. In the Houston study, however, there was one patient who had ocular hypertension preoperatively and had a marked steroid response, requiring treatment postoperatively. There have been several more patients who have had a rise of intraocular pressure postoperatively apparently as a response to topical steroids but which reduced with cessation of the steroids.

Endothelial Cell Loss. Sato's early radial keratotomy procedures resulted in significant endothelial cell loss.[13-16] It is believed that since radial keratotomy is now done without entering the anterior chamber and without intentionally incising Descemet's membrane, there should be minimal problem with endothelial cell loss. Studies have not shown consistent ongoing significant endothelial cell loss from modern anterior radial keratotomy (Table 13-1). However, there is always the risk of endothelial cell loss, especially in cases of corneal perforation. The role of indentation of the cornea resulting in increased endothelial cell loss has been discussed and investigated.[1] The final verdict is still not in, but significant endothelial cell loss from radial keratotomy does not appear to be a frequent complication. Cell density decrease may also not be due to cell destruction but rather to an increase in corneal surface area post-radial keratotomy.

Iron Line. Many surgeons see a small corneal iron line (Figure 13-24) just inferior to the optical axis frequently develop six to twelve months

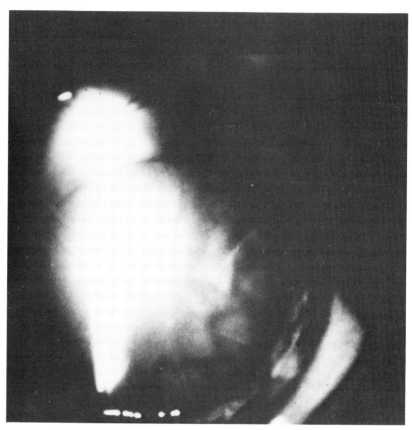

Figure 13-22. Clinical photograph of post-radial keratotomy cataract-etiology unknown. (Courtesy H. Gelender, M.D.)

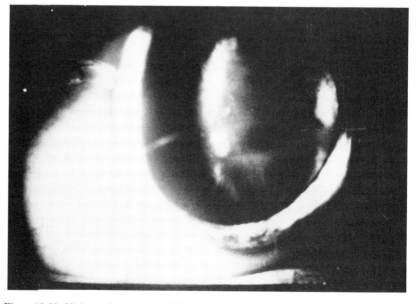

Figure 13-23. Slit lamp view of post-radial keratotomy cataract of unknown etiology. (Courtesy H. Gelender, M.D.)

TABLE 13-1

AUTHOR	COMMENT	% CELL CHANGE	FOLLOW-UP	DATE
Hoffer, Et Al.	16 Incisions	−9%	3 Months	Jun 83
Hoffer, Et Al.	16 Incisions	+2%	2 Years	Jun 83
Hoffer, Et Al.	8 Incisions	−2.6%	6 Months	Jun 83
Kremer & Marks	19 Cases	−4.5%	—	Nov 83
Rowsey & Balyeat		−6.5%	1 Month	Jan 82
Rowsey & Balyeat		−6.9%	6 Months	Jan 82
Rowsey & Balyeat	Cases c̄ perforation	−4.6%	1 Month	Jan 82
Rowsey & Balyeat	Cases c̄ perforation	−1%	6 Months	Jan 82
Rowsey & Balyeat	Pts c̄ fluctuation of	−9.4%	1 Month	Jan 82
Rowsey & Balyeat	vision	−15.7%	6 Months	Jan 82
Salz	One case: 5 Surgeries	−24%	14 Months	Dec 82
Rowsey & Balyeat	8 Patients	−4.5%	1 Year	Apr 82
Rowsey & Balyeat	Pts c̄ fluctuation of vision	−7.3%	>1 Year	Apr 82
Bores		−4.0		1983
Bores		−6.3		1983
Bores		−3.1		1983
Cowden	41 Patients	−0.62		1982

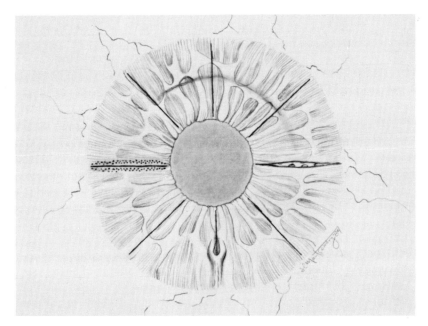

Figure 13-24. Mutiple slit lamp epithelial and subtle stromal opacities are seen post-radial keratotomy. Peri-incisional punctate epithelial keratopathy is frequently a harbinger of the leaking epithelial syndrome. Epithelial map lines or hair follicle shaped irregularities are found near midperipheral epithelial dragging sites due to surgical trauma. Iron lines are seen in approximately one-fourth of radial keratotomy patients later than one year. These iron lines have no adverse effects. Stromal incisional cysts are due to debris, epithelial cells, or wound healing difficulties.

postoperatively. Schachar has reported a rate of 10%[3] with other reports being as high as 33%. The authors have noted this iron line in 20% to 30% of cases over one year postoperatively; this epithelial iron line does not seem to have any adverse effect.

Recurrent Erosions. Recurrent erosions are a frequently reported complication, especially in patients 35 or older, but are not described as producing significant problems in management.[1] Minimizing epithelial trauma during surgery is important in avoiding recurrent erosions postoperatively. Patients who have recurrent erosions or punctate epithelial erosions should get aggressive treatment with ocular lubricants to aid epithelial healing. One patient seen in consultation in the Houston study was a 28-year-old patient two years postoperative who has had numerous erosions in an eye primarily operated upon with a steel blade and re-operated upon in the same incisions. She has numerous incisional cysts and the erosions usually occur over one of the cysts. This is the only experience with chronic recurrent epithelial erosions postoperatively in the Houston study.

Corneal Incision Cysts. Incisional cysts are generally seen in three situations: re-operations with cutting into previous incisions, use of steel blades, and debris left in incisions during surgery. The cysts are most commonly seen in re-operation patients where the re-operative incision followed or closely followed the original incisions. Cysts are larger and more common in patients operated upon using steel blades. Their cosmetic slit lamp appearance seems to have little clinical significance. Since much less scarring and/or cysts occur with a diamond blade, we generally make new virgin incisions with the diamond blade if an adjustment is needed. Cysts due to inclusional debris are further decreased (virtually never seen now) by careful irrigation of incisions. Nevertheless, take care *not* to irrigate into an incision with a microperforation.

Epithelial Dystrophy. The authors have encountered one case of exacerbation of corneal epithelium (map-dot) dystrophy from radial keratotomy with severe symptoms developing in the patient. The surgeon should be very careful to check for a history of corneal problems including recurrent erosions and family history of corneal problems. The history of problems with contact lens wear intolerance, reduced wearing time, or recurrent abrasions should alert the surgeon to the possibility of epithelial dystrophy. During initial examination it is important to look for subtle evidence of corneal epithelial dystrophy including reduplications of Bowman's membrane with Cogan's dystrophy and epithelial microcysts of Meesman's dystrophy. In older patients and those with a higher number of incisions, a central corneal epithelial defect may develop in the acute postoperative period. These defects generally re-epithelialize within two to three days without consequence. These defects can be treated with patching and/or artificial tears. No lubricating ointment should be used in the immediate postoperative course to avoid petrolatum debris from entering the incisions.

Endothelial Dystrophy. Corneal guttata carry a double risk: possible increased endothelial cell loss from surgery resulting in corneal decompensation and the tendency for these corneas to grossly overcorrect. These patients should be discouraged from having incisional refractive keratoplasty.

Keratoconus. Radial keratotomy which flattens the central cornea would *seem* to be the perfect extraocular treatment of keratoconus with its excessively steep central cornea. However, keratoconus patients get very unpredictable results from radial keratotomy. Another problem in keratoconus with radial keratotomy is the development of a heavy proliferation of scar tissue into the stroma surrounding the incisions. This proliferation can especially be a problem if subclinical or formes fruste of keratoconus are not diagnosed. Large amounts of astigmatism and/or very steep keratometry readings, especially over 48 diopters, should alert the surgeon to the possibility of keratoconus. Careful examination may reveal other signs of keratoconus. Photokeratoscopy may be helpful preoperatively to diagnose subtle cases of keratoconus. The authors have had some keratoconus patients get an improvement in their best corrected visual acuity through reduction of their astigmatism using a Ruiz procedure. One patient went from 20/60 best corrected to 20/40 uncorrected, with best correction to 20/25. In the preoperative discussion the uncertainty of the operation on the keratoconus cornea must be heavily emphasized and other treatment forms presented.

References

1. Schachar RA: *Understanding Radial Keratotomy,* Denison, TX: LAL Publishing, 1981.
2. Sanders DR, (ed): *Radial Keratotomy.* Thorofare, NJ: Slack, Inc., 1984.
3. Schachar RA: "Indications, Techniques, and Complications of Radial Keratotomy." *In* Binder P (ed), *Refractive Corneal Surgery: The Correction of Aphakia, Hyperopia, and Myopia.* International Ophthalmology Clinics, Vol 23, No 3, 1983. Boston, MA: Little, Brown and Co., 1983, pp 112-128.
4. Villaseñor RA, et al: Changes in Corneal Thickness During Radial Keratotomy. *Ophth Surg* 12(5):341, 1981.
5. Arrowsmith PN, et al: Visual, Refractive and Keratometric Results of Radial Keratotomy. *Arch Ophth* 101:837, 1983.
6. Gelender H, Parel J: Vacuum Fixation Ring for Radial Keratotomy. *Ophth Surg* 15:(2):126-126, 1984.
7. Gelender H, Flynn HW, Mendelbaum SH: Bacterial Endophthalmitis Following Radial Keratotomy. *Am J Ophth* 93:323, 1982.
8. Rylander HG, Welch AJ, Fremming B: The Effect of Radial Keratotomy on the Rupture Strength of Pig Eyes. *Ophth Surg* 14(9):744-749, 1983.
9. Larson BC, Kremer FB, Eller AW, Bernardino VB: Quantitated Trauma Following Radial Keratotomy in Rabbits. *Ophthalmology* 90(6):660-667, 1983.
10. John ME, Schmitt TE: Traumatic Hyphema After Radial Keratotomy. *Ann Ophthalmol* 15(10):930-932, 1983.
11. Baldone JA, Franklin RM: Cataract Following Radial Keratotomy. *Ann Ophthalmol* 15(5):416-418, 1983.
12. Schachar RA: *Refractive Keratoplasty,* Denison, TX: LAL Publishing, 1983.
13. Bores LD: "Historical Review and Clinical Results of Radial Keratotomy." *in* PS Binder (ed) *Refractive Corneal Surgery: The Correction of Aphakia, Hyperopia, and Myopia.* International Ophthalmology Clinics Vol. 23, No. 3, 1983. Boston, MA: Little, Brown and Co. 1983, pp 93-128.
14. Cowden JJ, Sultana M: Corneal Endothelial Cell Density Following Radial Keratotomy. *Invest Ophthalmol Vis Sci* (Suppl) 22(3):30, 1982.

15. Salz JJ: Progressive Endothelial Cell Loss Following Repeat Radial Keratotomy—A Case Report *Ophth Surg* 13(12):997-999, 1982.
16. Akiyama K, Tanaka M, Kanai A, Nakajima A: Problems Arising from Sato's Radial Keratotomy Procedure in Japan *CLAO J* 10(2):179-184, 1984.

Chapter 14

Radial Keratotomy: Results and Complications

William Myers, MD

RADIAL KERATOTOMY: RESULTS AND COMPLICATIONS

During the last 10 years ophthalmic clinicians have become much more critical in their evaluations of reported clinical data. In all probability the experience with intraocular lenses has sensitized them to the importance of such issues as long-term follow up, surgeon bias, acceptable experimental designs, and other factors which make the results of a given study more or less credible. The purpose of this chapter is to critically review some of the reported results and complications of radial keratotomy and to draw some conclusions concerning the status of this procedure.

The initial report of Sato is of value, not because of what it tells us about radial keratotomy, but because of what it indicates about the importance of long-term results and losses to follow up. Sato's initial results indicated that his technique, which utilized anterior and posterior corneal surface incisions, was safe and effective in correcting small amounts of myopia.[1] However, the more recent literature and other reports have shown that this procedure resulted in postsurgical corneal edema and bullous keratopathy. Obviously, the acceptance of only the short-term results and inadequate follow up of individuals who ultimately developed a keratopathy would have given a falsely optimistic impression of the Sato procedure.

Fyodorov, the one most responsible for the development of radial keratotomy, provided the first clinical data to appear in the American ophthalmic literature.[2] His early reports were remarkable not only in the apparent effectiveness of the procedure, but also in the apparent lack of reported complications. Subsequent to the appearance of these reports in American literature, Fyodorov had shared with many of his American colleagues a few rare cases of postoperative keratopathy and neovascularization. These observations are not a criticism of Fyodorov's early data since we have discovered he was indeed generally accurate with his conclusions concerning the efficacy and relative safety of radial keratotomy; they merely point out, once again, the importance of guarding against having patients lost to follow up.

Bores, the first American surgeon to perform radial keratotomy, reported on the American results in 1981.[3] The results correlated fairly well with those of Fyodorov. Bores found that in his series of 303 eyes, 61% achieved an acuity of 20/40 or better. He reported no serious surgical complications. He also reported an endothelial cell loss of 6.3%. The pioneering efforts of Fyodorov and Bores were viewed with caution by other ophthalmologists. Such early findings, of course, required confirmation by other individuals in order to enhance their credibility. Such confirmative reports were soon forthcoming.

Table 14-1
Summary Statistics of Six Reported Series of Radial Keratotomy Surgeries

	Hoffer et al[4]	Hoffer et al[4]	Nirankiri et al[5]	Arrowsmith et al[6]	Deitz et al[7]	Thornton[8] #
No. of Eyes	80	62	58	156	290	200
Avg. Preop Myopia	−5.2	−3.8	−4.6	−5.0	−4.8	−5.25
Range of Myopia						
Minimum	−2.0	−2.0	−1.75	−1.5	−0.9	−2.0
Maximum	−13.5	−6.75	−12.25	−16.0	−10.3	−18.5
% Follow-up (period)	65% (2 yr)	100% (2 yr)	100% (6 mo)	89% (9 mo)	93% (1 yr)	94% (1 yr)
Preop VA >20/400	54%	23%	14%	51%	65%	71%
Avg. Incision Depth	*	*	50%	*	90%	85%
No. of Incisions	16	8	8-16	8-16	8-16	8-16
Peripheral Redeepening	Yes	No	No	Yes	No	Yes
PostOp Uncorrected VA						
20/20	36%	28%	12%	43%	40%	43%
<20/40	50%	65%	48%	73%	83%	73%
Low/Moderate Myopes	(<5D)	(<6.75D)	(<5D)	(<6D)	(<6D)	(<5D)
20/20	50%	28%	13%	53%	46%	60%
<20/40	69%	65%	63%	84%	88%	75%
Avg. Myopia Correction	3.8D	2.8D	2.7D	5.0D	5.0D	*
% Within 1D of Emmetropia	*	*	29%	51%	60%	75%
Overcorrection >2D	6%	0	*	14%	6%	2%
Reoperations	*	*	10%	8%	0.6%	4%
Microperforations	19%	0	0	35%	37%	~8%

(*) Data not available in published reports.
(#) Further information was obtained from author since series was not reported in referred journal.

Results

Table 14-1 summarizes six reported series of radial keratotomy surgeries. While these are not the only reported series, they all had independent evaluations; they studied a reasonably large number of cases; and they reported their data in a sufficiently similar format to allow comparison of their results.

The average amount of myopia corrected varied between 2.7 and 5.0 diopters, depending on the series. With the exception of the series by Nirankari et al, where the incisions were reported to be too shallow (50% depth), overall postoperative uncorrected visual acuity was 20/20 in 28% to 43% of cases, and it was 20/40 or better in 50% to 83% of cases. In patients with preoperative refractive errors of 5 to 6 diopters or less, as many as 46% to 60% of patients attained 20/20 uncorrected acuity, and in at least two series, more than 80% achieved 20/40 vision or better.

My own initial series of 400 radial keratotomy patients, first reported in 1981, correlated quite well with the early results of other surgeons. Seventy-three percent of all patients had postoperative uncorrected visual acuities of 20/40 or better. The breakdown of the postoperative visual results is shown in Table 14-2. The patients' preoperative refractive errors ranged from −1.50 diopters to −18.0 diopters with a mean of −5.5 diopters. There was, of course, a correlation between the degree of preoperative myopia and the resultant uncorrected postoperative visual acuities. Seventy-eight percent of 259 eyes with refractive errors of 6.0 diopters or less had postoperative acuities of 20/40 or better. For cases with 5.25 diopters or less, the percentage achieving 20/40 or better increased to 81%. The complications in this series, which are shown in Table 14-3, were generally caused by imperfect surgical technique or the fitting of soft lenses in the early postoperative phase.

Since the time of this early series, the ability to make uniformly deep

---

Table 14-2
Postoperative Visual Acuity—First 400 Patients

Uncorrected Visual Acuity Postoperatively	Number of Patients	Percentage	
20/20	56	14	
20/25	56	14	
20/30	88	22	
20/40	92	23	
	Subtotal		73
20/50-20/100	48	12	
20/200 or less	60	15	
	Subtotal		27

Table 14-3
Complications of First 400 Cases

Complication	Number
Micro-perforations	3
Macro-perforations	0
Recurrent Erosions	0
Infections	0
Induced Cylinder (0.50-1.00 D)	19
Irregular Astigmatism	3
Reduction in Best Corrected Acuity	2
Neovascularization	4

Table 14-4
Postoperative Visual Acuity—Last 400 Patients

Uncorrected Visual Acuity Postoperatively	Number of Patients	Percentage	
20/20 or better	192	48	
20/25	56	14	
20/30	52	13	
20/40	44	11	
	Subtotal		86
20/50-20/100	32	8	
20/200 or less	24	6	
	Subtotal		14

incisions has improved due to the perfection of diamond micrometer knives and integrated gauge blocks. A review of my last 400 cases shows how these advances in instrumentation have positively influenced the results. As Table 14-4 indicates, 86% of the patients in this latter series achieved uncorrected postoperative visual acuities of 20/40 or better. The only complications in this series of 400 cases were seven eyes having a small induced cylinder.

Complications

The following complications are known to be associated with radial keratotomy, as evidenced by the findings of multiple surgeons. A more complete discussion of the complications of radial keratotomy is given in Chapter 20.

Perforations. In a series of over 1,000 cases, I have had a total of six perforations. These perforations have all been microperforations, requiring no suture and having no loss of the anterior chamber. These microperforations had no effect on the course of the operation or the postoperative results. An example of a macroperforation, which requires a suture in order to maintain the anterior chamber, is shown in Figure 14-1. At least one case of endophthalmitis has occurred in a radial keratotomy case in which a perforation was noted operatively. Even this single event emphasizes the obvious fact that we should attempt to avoid significant perforations whenever possible. This is best achieved by adopting a technique which allows constant visualization of the tip of the diamond knife while incising in a slow and deliberate manner. In this way, the surgeon can note a microperforation and discontinue the cut before a macroperforation occurs.

Neovascularization. In 1981 I first noted first case of neovascularization following radial keratotomy (Figure 14-2). This patient was not fully corrected and was fitted with a soft lens approximately two months postoperatively. This patient also had radial keratotomy incisions which extended to the vascular arcades of the limbus. This complication is avoided either by keeping incisions at least 1 mm away from the limbovascular arcades or by not fitting the patient with a soft lens until the K-readings and refraction are stable. An extreme degree of neovascularization, as reported by Fyodorov, is shown in Figure 14-3.

Overcorrections. Only a small number of my patients have achieved postoperative hyperopia requiring glasses or contact lenses. However, I have seen in consultation one patient with a preoperative refraction of −4.00 diopters who postoperatively developed +6.00 diopters of hyper-

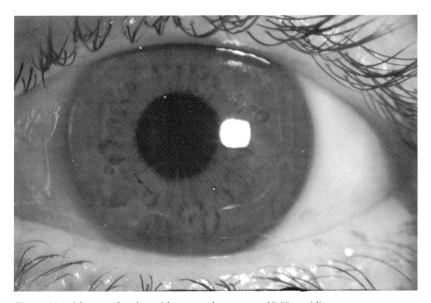

Figure 14-1. Macroperforation with suture placement at 10:00 meridian.

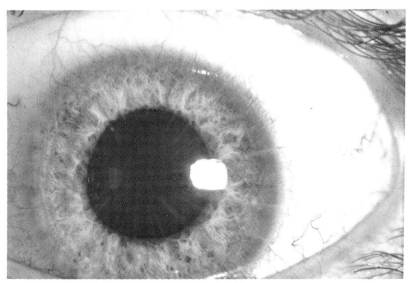

Figure 14-2. Early neovascularization due to premature soft lens fitting following radial keratotomy.

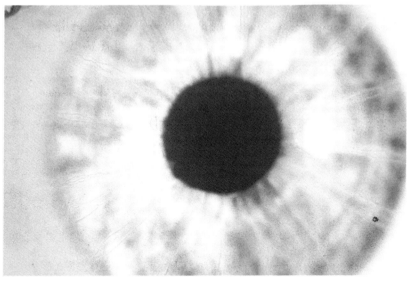

Figure 14-3. Extensive neovascularization following radial keratotomy.

opia which did not regress. The patient's fellow unoperated eye had −4.00 diopters of myopia. His postoperative corneal curvature was so flat that a properly fitting contact lens was not possible. To alleviate his extreme anisometropia he underwent an onlay-graft by Dr. Marguerite MacDonald at Louisiana State University. His appearance in the early postoperative phase following the onlay-graft is shown in Figure 14-4.

Significant overcorrections generally occur in individuals who are in

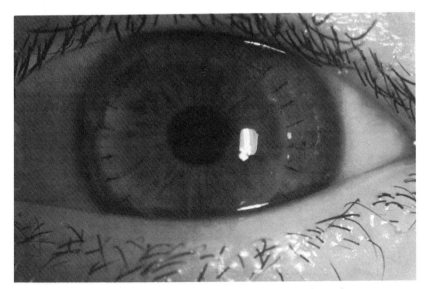

Figure 14-4. Treatment of radial keratotomy overcorrection with onlay-graft.

their late 30's and older with mild to moderate amounts of myopia. I now approach such patients by using a four-incision radial keratotomy This approach is most helpful in avoiding overcorrections while allowing the surgeon the option of correcting any residual myopia with a second series of four incisions. In cases in which a four-incision radial keratotomy has been performed, I found that the four incisions achieved approximately 67% of the effect one would anticipate if eight incisions had been utilized with the same size of optical zone.

Undercorrections. Residual myopia is present in approximately 10% to 20% of radial keratotomy patients, depending on the series under review. Most of the patients in this group are in their late 20's or younger with higher amounts of preoperative myopia. Along with patient selection, the depth of the incisions is closely related to the problem of undercorrection. If the incision is less than 90% of the total corneal thickness, the possibility of an undercorrection increases.

Glare. Glare in the early postoperative period is a phenomenon that almost all radial keratotomy patients experience. Only when it persists after several months should it be classified as a true complication. Unquestionably, glare can be produced by incisions which migrate into the zone of the pupil. Surgical error with regard to the centration of the optical zone can be one of the causes. Individual cuts extending into the optical zone can also result in glare. This latter complication, shown in Figure 14-5, can best be avoided by making the cuts from the optical zone toward the limbus and not in the reverse direction, as advocated by some radial keratotomy surgeons.

Glare can also be produced by radial keratotomy scars that are excessively thick. Thickened scars are generally produced by repeated keratot-

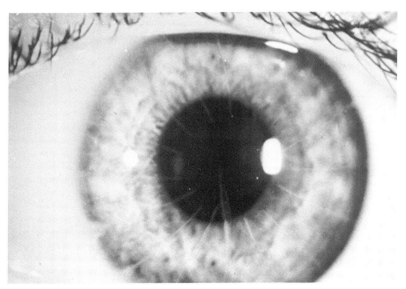

Figure 14-5. Incursion of incision into optical zone at 6:00 meridian.

omy incisions. Scars can occur in an original surgical procedure which utilizes redeepening of the incisions if redeepening is not carried out in the same surgical plane as the initial incision. Thick scars can also occur in repeat radial keratotomy incisions in which the surgeon attempts to re-enter the original corneal scars, which is generally a very difficult proposition at best. An example of a patient who underwent a redeepening procedure in the initial surgery with subsequent scarring is shown in Figure 14-6. It is also important to realize that some patients will be bothered by glare even though the procedure was perfectly done. For this reason it is important that glare be mentioned during the course of informing the patient. For those with objectionable glare, 0.5% pilocarpine can be helpful, especially at night.

Fluctuating Vision. Fluctuating vision, like glare, is present in all cases during the initial postoperative stage. It disappears after several months in the vast majority of patients. In patients in whom the fluctuating vision is bothersome, a pair of glasses for night driving is generally required.

Recurrent Erosions. Some radial keratotomy patients describe symptoms which are compatible with small recurrent erosions. This is a diagnosis that is frequently made by history because at the time of examination, the patient's epithelial surface looks totally intact. Generally these patients will be in the older age groups. The use of Lacri-Lube at bedtime is effective in these cases.

Iron Deposits. Careful biomicroscopy demonstrates iron lines in approximately 20% of all radial keratotomy patients. Surface irregularities during the postoperative period are probably responsible for this finding.

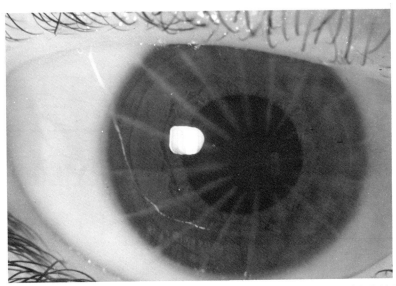

Figure 14-6. Thick radial keratotomy scars following a secondary redeepening of the initial surgical incisions.

Summary

The initial reports of both Fyodorov and Bores indicated that radial keratotomy was effective in reducing myopia with a degree of safety compatible with its use in individuals with normal corneas. The results of numerous other surgeons, many of whom have been cited in this chapter, support their conclusions.

References

1. Sato T, Akiyama K, Shibata H: A New Surgical Approach to Myopia. *Am J of Ophthalmol* 36:823-829, 1953.
2. Fyodorov S, Durnev V: Operation of Dosage Dissection of Corneal Circular Ligament in Cases of Myopia of Mild Degree. *Ann Ophthalmol* 11:1855-1889, 1979.
3. Bores L, Myers W, Cowden J: Radial Keratotomy: An analysis of the American experience. *Ann Ophthalmol* 13:941-948, 1981.
4. Hoffer K, Darin J, Pettit T, Hofbauer J, Elander R, Levenson J: Three Year Experience with Radial Keratotomy: The UCLA study. *Ophthalmol* 90:627-636, 1983.
5. Narankiri V, Katzen L, Karesh J, Richards R, Lakhanpal V: Ongoing Prospective Clinical Study in Radial Keratotomy. *Ophthalmology* 90:637-641, 1983.
6. Arrowsmith P, Sanders D, Marks R: Visual, Refractive, and Keratometric Results of Radial Keratotomy. *Arch Ophthalmol* 101:873-881, 1983.
7. Deitz M, Sanders D, Marks R: Radial Keratotomy: An overview of the Kansas City study. *Ophthalmology* 91:467-478, 1983.
8. DeBenedette V: High Success Rate Reported in Radial Keratotomy Series. *Ophthalmol Times* 8:18, 1983.